HERE IS WHAT THEY ARE SAYING:

"Thanks for saving my sex life." — *J.E. (Post-Partum Pelvic Pain)*

"Ending Female Pain is a treasure. Isa Herrera has put together the best possible resource for helping women heal pelvic pain and live fully and comfortably."

> — *Christiane Northrup, MD, ob/gyn physician and author of the New York Times bestsellers: Women's Bodies, Women's Wisdom and The Wisdom of Menopause*

"A breakthrough for women... this book is the ultimate self-healing resource for chronic pelvic pain and post-partum complications."

> — *Ricki Lake and Abby Epstein, filmmakers of "The Business of Being Born" and authors of "Your Best Birth"*

"Before I started doing Isa's exercises the pain was so severe I couldn't even sit."

> — *D.P. NYC (Interstitial Cystitis and Pelvic Pain)*

"My patients recover faster and have less pain after doing Isa's exercises and receiving her unique treatments. Hands down she is the best in NYC."

> — *Jacques Moritz, MD, OB/GYN in NYC*

"The homework, exercises and treatment that Isa gave me helped me. Today I am pain free." — *K.J.C. (Pelvic Pain)*

"Isa proved to be my secret weapon against vestibulodynia. She has made it her life's work to understand how to unlock the body to lessen the grip of vaginal pain. Isa got me ready both physically and psychologically to face the frightening realities of a vestibulectomy. Whenever I would get discouraged, she would help me build up my mental framework and shore me up against the frustrations of this very mentally-challenging disease."

> — *J. Q. (Vestibulitis & Post-Surgical Vestibulectomy Patient)*

ENDING
female
PAIN

A Woman's Manual

ENDING
fema/e
PAIN

A Woman's Manual

*The Ultimate Self-Help Guide for Women
Suffering from Chronic Pelvic and Sexual Pain*

ISA HERRERA
MSPT, CSCS

Published in the United States by Duplex Publishing, New York.

1st printing-October 2009. 2nd printing April 2010.

10 Digit ISBN: 1-4392-5777-9

13 Digit EAN: 978-1-4392-5777-7

Maria Paz Cabardo – Design

David Ondrick – Digital production and Project management

Maria Rosario Gallegos – Proofreading and Editing

Richard Simpson – Photographer

Winston Johnson – Illustrations

Acknowledgements

Ella Jade Audrey Ondrick for being Ella, my wonderful daughter; Solange Leitner – Model and great women's health physical therapist; Nancy Salicrup for hair and makeup; Zoe Bowick Levine and Charlotte Blake – Personal trainer and Exercise specialists; Dr. Jacques Moritz for his insightful foreword; Rosita Arvigo, Kathe Wallace, Holly Herman, Elizabeth Noble, Dr. Elaine Rosen, and Dr. Martha Sliwinski for inspiration; Amy Slotnick for guidance and direction; Rosie Pineda for being there from day one; my mom Crucita for being mom; and Ricki Lake and Abby Epstein for helping increase awareness on the topic of women's health.

Medical Disclaimer

The information in this book is not meant as a substitute for healthcare. Consult your healthcare provider for a complete check-up because pelvic pain can be the result of a serious medical condition or medical pathology.

Most patients need a multi-layered approach to overcome their chronic pelvic pain. Make sure to see doctors and specialists in the field of female sexual pain and pelvic floor muscle dysfunction, and then talk to your doctor about getting a referral to a physical therapist that specializes in pelvic floor muscle dysfunction. It is also extremely important to educate yourself about your pelvic pain condition. Do not be afraid to ask questions of your caregivers, or to get a second opinion about your condition.

This book would not have been possible without the love and endless support of my husband David and my daughter Ella. I dedicate this book to them and to all my female patients who motivate me to think outside the box to fine-tune the tools and mind-body techniques in this book. Their stories and firm resolve to end their pain continue to fuel my search for answers.

Contents

Foreword

by Dr. Jacques Moritz

Director of Obstetrics and Gynecology Division, St. Luke's Roosevelt Hospital

In my over 15 years of work at St. Luke's, I have seen women from all walks of life who experience sexual pain or some other type of pelvic disorder. More often than not, these women end up suffering quietly because they are told that the pain is in their heads. They quickly give up, unaware that there are remedies to get them back to normal.

Doctors are often ignorant of these remedies because they are not trained in medical school in ways to deal with post-operative, post-delivery or generalized vulvar pain, much less pain during sexual intercourse. Sadly, many women are also brought up to accept pelvic pain as part of their lives.

Although pelvic health and rehabilitation is a critical part of female wellness, it is often the most neglected aspect of their care in this country. I believe the main reason for this neglect is because no one wants to deal with or talk about pain in a woman's vagina. After a woman has a baby, a pelvic surgery, or experiences painful intercourse, often no effort is made to eliminate the pain or to test whether her pelvic floor muscles function properly. In other countries like France, for example, pelvic rehabilitation is considered an integral part of the healing process post-childbirth and pelvic surgery. It only makes sense to treat trauma to a very delicate area the same way a broken leg requires therapy.

The first thing women need to know is that the pain is not in their heads. Pelvic pain is not a normal part of life, that sex is supposed to be pleasurable, and if there is pain, it is a sign that something is wrong. If your current doctor does not believe in this philosophy there are three things you can do to help yourself. One, find a doctor that understands this philosophy. Two, while your doctor understands this philosophy, you also need to understand that pelvic pain is a source of frustration to them because they are not trained to deal with this. Three, seek out a physical therapist who specializes in pelvic floor muscle rehabilitation. In the United States, doctors do not routinely recommend this type of rehabilitation, causing women to suffer needlessly. That is why this book is so important for women everywhere.

It must also be known that there are no quick fixes for pelvic pain; there isn't a cream, gel, or an exercise that is going to fix it. It is going to be a series of trials and errors but it can be done. Frustration will make the situation worse than when it started. Isa has taken an interest where most physical therapists do not even want to deal with – a field that most find is not for them. She listens to women, is responsive, understands their pain, and does everything in her power to rehabilitate them. She is also realistic and understands her patients are not always going to end up with zero pain, but she always tries everything in her arsenal of tools to help women avoid unnecessary surgeries.

Ending Female Pain is the most complete resource on the market that offers women self-help treatment from pains caused by childbirth trauma, scar pains from abdominal surgeries, and chronic pelvic and sexual pain, empowering them to overcome their pain themselves. Isa has a unique talent. She is very committed to teaching her patients to break their cycles of pain, whether psychologically or with physical therapy, or both. She believes that hope of recovery lies with her patients and puts them on the path to getting better themselves. In *Ending Female Pain,* Isa gives you the proven strategies and unique techniques that have brought relief to countless numbers of her patients – precisely the information that women need to restore their sexual and day-to-day function, and that is why I highly recommend this book.

Part 1
OVERVIEW

"A jar fills drop by drop."
— Buddha

Chapter 1

INTRODUCTION

How does one get involved in my line of work? This is a question I am often asked by my patients. As I have come to realize, I always knew I wanted to be involved with women's health. My experiences in the last ten years – first as a fitness instructor and now as a physiotherapist - have shaped my vision of care and empowerment. After hearing the stories of my patients, I have decided to write a self-help manual for the relief of sexual pain based on the various treatments I have given them.

My first exposure to pelvic floor muscle dysfunction came when I taught pre- and post-natal exercise classes in New York City. I was always interested in the things my students told me about the pain they were feeling. Hearing the things these women had to say and what they were going through piqued my interest, but as a pre- and post-natal fitness instructor I lacked the tools and knowledge to help these women on such a complex level. They would tell me things like, "After I had my baby it hurts every time I have sex"; "After the baby came, my husband no longer fits inside me"; "My episiotomy scar opens up after sex"; or "I've never been comfortable having sex at all." I am here to tell you not to be afraid to talk about these issues, because they are common threads among women I have treated and are not spoken about freely enough in the community.

I know now that these problems can be grouped under blanket terms like vulvodynia, dyspareunia, vaginismus, and perineal pain. Many of their complaints are related to pelvic floor muscle (PFM) dysfunctions such as incoordination, spasms, muscle hypertonicity, muscle shortness, trigger points and scar adhesions. Hearing their stories and trying to answer their questions about why they were in pain inspired me to embark on a quest for answers to end female pain. After the birth of my own child, things just didn't feel right down there. And then after a yeast infection and several bouts of antibiotics, not only did sex hurt but now my vulva would burn with a constant ache. After my own personal experience with sexual pain, and after hearing countless stories of other women's bouts with chronic pelvic pain, I decided to make it my life's mission to help women heal their pelvic pain conditions.

At first I found no single resource out there to free myself from vaginal discomfort and pain, so I started to educate myself on PFM dysfunction. I studied with the best teachers, shadowed many doctors in their practices, took countless courses on the topic of PFM dysfunction, and finished my Masters in Physical Therapy. I decided that the best way to help my patients was to create a central source from which they could identify their conditions and empower themselves to overcome their pain. After several years of toil, I was able to open my own healing center in New York City, which I call Renew Physical Therapy.

At my healing center, I give the women under my care many different tools, exercises and techniques to use at home, which I collectively call "The Renew Program For Women™." Many find complete relief with my treatments and unique protocols, and some experience life-changing relief from their chronic pain. To see what some of my graduates have to say, visit my website at *www.Renew-PT.com* and view the video testimonials. This book, *Ending Female Pain*, is the next step in bringing my message out to a wider audience by incorporating all of my experiences into an easy-to-read woman's manual.

I've had many successes in treating women with sexual pain, and I must say that the women who are the most successful either possess or develop a positive fighting attitude and learn how to take control of their pain on their own. Taking control is not easy, but by incorporating the tools in my book you can give yourself the momentum to get the ball rolling.

When I tell people what I do for a living I often receive blank stares. Many people have either never heard of PFM dysfunction or painful sex or have never had any exposure to conditions that involve pelvic floor muscles such as interstitial cystitis, dyspareunia, vaginismus, lichen sclerosus and many more. And why would they know about these medical conditions that create havoc on women's lives? Most women enjoy sex, have no pain with penetration, have no lingering burning after orgasms, have no vulvar pain with sitting, and have no discomfort with tight clothes rubbing on their private parts. Some do not even experience any painful symptoms after childbirth. This book is written for the woman who has experienced some or all of the above symptoms, and especially for the woman who has been told things like, "There is nothing wrong" or "The pain is in your head" or "Things like that can happen."

My approach in *Ending Female Pain* is a comprehensive and empowering one. The focus is on the whole person with exercises for both mind and body. Have you ever heard the expression "It takes a village"? That's exactly how I feel about caring for women with chronic pelvic pain. Chronic pelvic pain is a complex medical condition requiring, in my opinion, a multidisciplinary medical and holistic mind-body approach. Women will have to incorporate many different treatments to help resolve their pelvic pain, and they should also know that there are other women who are experiencing the same feelings and discomforts. With this book, I hope to increase the level of dialogue and end the silent suffering of so many women out there.

If you are currently suffering from sexual pain, you will have to give up the notion that you will never get better and that this is the way things will remain. This kind of catastrophic thinking will only hinder your healing process. As you go through this book, try out all the exercises and techniques and select those that work for you. At times you may say, "These techniques don't work for me," and then you might come back a few weeks later to try them again and find that they give you great pain relief. Always keep an open mind when working with the tools in this book. Remember, every day is different. Your body will respond differently on different days.

I give my patients a lot of homework and tell them that their treatment consists of physical therapy plus independent study. You will have to put yourself first on your own list in order to heal yourself. Don't say things like, "I'm too tired tonight to do my own self-healing work." Instead, put aside all your doubts and fears, and decide to become your own savior.

I encourage you to be proactive in your own healing journey and to seek practitioners who will partner with you in your healthcare. Partnership healthcare is the only way to go. Work with caregivers who specialize in the field of pelvic pain and always follow your instincts when choosing your healthcare team. You must trust and believe in them. Select caregivers who have an open mind and are willing to try different methods, techniques, medicines and technologies to get you better. Make sure they take the time to hear what you are saying and feeling, and be sure they answer your questions no matter how trivial they may seem.

Most importantly, you must keep your head up and avoid negative self-talk. Never give up on yourself. Search for your answers with intelligence and sensibility. Always follow your own heart and intuition. If something doesn't feel right or hurts, that's an internal cue to stop and listen to your body. Do not ignore what your body is telling you.

This concept of listening to your body is especially true when you perform many of the exercises and techniques in this book. If it hurts, stop, reassess and ask yourself if this technique or exercise is the right one for you. Ask: "Am I being too aggressive with the tools? If I do this technique gently and slowly, will it hurt less and give me pain relief?" Oftentimes, the techniques you try will cause some pain as you take back control of your body, but just remember to listen to the messages your body is telling you.

Keep track of the tools and exercises that you do and become your own expert on what helps to relieve your pelvic pain. Understand that when you use the tools in this book you will have setbacks. At times, you may experience more pain. This is normal. Wait a few days and see how you feel. If symptoms flare up due to the exercises, you may feel worse for 24 to 72 hours, but eventually, you will feel better. It's the same as when you work out at the gym. There's always muscle soreness.

Now that I have covered the overall background to my mission and have primed you to get started, remember that ultimately you hold the key to your own healing. Go through this book carefully and with an open mind. You have two roads to choose from: the road to eliminate your own sexual pain or the road to stay as you are and do nothing. Read *Ending Female Pain* and make yourself the heroine of your own story.

Chapter Two

*"I am not discouraged, because
every wrong attempt discarded
is another step forward."*
—Thomas Edison

Chapter 2

HOW TO USE THIS BOOK

In this book I share my trade secrets to put you on the road to a pain-free and wonderful sex life. *Ending Female Pain* represents a fusion of exercises, pain-relief techniques, and body-mind methods that I've put together to help my patients defeat their pelvic pain. Working with patients suffering from pelvic pain, I discovered a core group of exercises and techniques, that when incorporated into my patients' self-care program, helped them reduce their pain, enabled them to sit longer, allowed them to function better, and ultimately gave them back their lives. These simple-to-learn and easy-to-implement techniques helped many of my patients get rid of their sexual pain. These techniques are rolled up into "The Renew Program For Women™."

The tools are a set of holistic, natural and non-surgical methods for the treatment of female chronic pelvic pain. This unique approach incorporates several protocols that I have developed, helping many of my patients enjoy pain-free sex again or for the first time.

The large selection of techniques in this book are based on the latest medical research and on my real-life, practical experience in treating patients. The techniques include deep and superficial massage, trigger point and myofascial release, internal vaginal stretching, external pelvic muscle stretching, myofascial foam rolling, relaxation exercises, breathing techniques, and others. Above all I consider myself a coach in the lives of my patients, carefully tailoring a holistic body and mind program that works for them.

You will find that after reading this book you will become an active participant in your own self-care and treatment. You will learn how to manage and control your pain on your own, and you will feel more hopeful in your journey. *Ending Female Pain*, with its innovative methods and scientifically-based exercises, will help put you on the right track to pain-free and wonderful sex. You will be able to perform your daily chores with ease, develop a more positive outlook, and realize there are ways that you can help yourself when you experience pelvic pain flare-ups. Overall, your quality of life will improve.

What I do is physiotherapy, and what I tell my patients is that they must participate physically, emotionally, and spiritually in their treatments in order to achieve their goal of pain-free intercourse. By teaching my patients specific exercise techniques, sexual healing methods, and behavioral changes, they learn to care for themselves with the knowledge that they need to be self-sufficient and in control of their pain. At first, many of my patients feel insecure about doing the exercises and techniques on their own, but like everything else, practice makes perfect.

Exercise alone will not set you on the road to pain-free sex. You must also address your mindset and perform mental hygiene on a daily basis. Mental hygiene is extremely important. I have observed that the women I treat who are suffering from chronic pelvic pain conditions tend to be depressed. They feel hopeless because their journey has been a difficult and trying one. Many chronic pelvic pain sufferers need help with stress reduction. Many need a renewal of their spirit and soul. I believe strongly that you are what you think. Adopting a more positive outlook will help put you on the road to full recovery.

Remember that many of the women I treat have suffered pelvic pain for years. Many have gone from doctor to doctor in search of answers. Many have been told it's all in their head, or even worse, have been told to relax or to grin and bear it. Without any relief to their pain, these women are left feeling anxious, depressed and hopeless. Because of the pain that having sex brings, many avoid intimate relations with their partners resulting in strained relationships. Many endure sex even though the pain is excruciating because they fear losing their men. Other women abstain from sex and avoid being in relationships, leading to loneliness and isolation. All these emotional experiences just accumulate and add to the suffering, depression, stress and anxiety they feel. These experiences lead to catastrophic thinking and result in negative behaviors. You are not alone. I want you to use this book as a springboard to realize that there are many other women out there who are feeling the same things as you. Throughout this book I have included stories from my patients so you can see that results are out there if you work hard enough. Here is a story from one of my patients.

In Their Own Words – Finding Relief for Painful Sex

"I've had pain with sexual intercourse for years. It has been greatly affecting my relationship, my personal happiness and self-esteem. I always felt like I was the only one out there with such a problem. It was really hard for me to talk to someone about it, even close friends.

"I've seen numerous gynecologists that couldn't help me at all. Physically they didn't find anything wrong with me so they didn't know what to do with my problem. I never felt really taken cared of or listened to.

"Finally I was referred to a pelvic pain specialist that did believe in my pain being real. I thought he would be the one to finally help me. After numerous tests he diagnosed me with interstitial cystitis (IC). I was put on a very expensive medication called Elmiron® that I had to pay for out of my own pocket since I don't have proper health insurance.

"Elmiron® is a medication that really impacts your daily life because of the way you have to coordinate it with your meals. Also, you are supposed to take it for at least 3 to 6 months to see any improvement. Needless to say I wasn't happy with it, but I gave it a chance.

"It helped with urinary frequency but I did not get any relief from the pain I felt with intercourse. I felt helpless and longed to find alternatives. So I researched and spoke to people and finally ended up at Renew Physical Therapy.

"I am thrilled that I found Isa and her team. They are welcoming, understanding and comforting. They even offered a great payment plan for the physical therapy (PT) program. After an initial exam, Isa found that I had very tight muscles and started treating me and teaching me internal and external exercises to do at home.

"My doctor had never been able to find these muscular 'spasms' and tight spots. He even said specifically that PT wouldn't help me. I am proud that I took the initiative and made him prescribe PT for me regardless. You just have to really see what options you have and not just blindly listen to what your doctor tells you.

"Isa has a gift, and she knows women's bodies inside out. She has a very holistic approach to her treatment which I love. She gave me tons of tips on relaxation, nutrition, exercising, etc. But the most important part is that she empowers women to help themselves. PT is not a miracle treatment. You have to do the work yourself in order to get better. But with Isa's help and understanding, I was able to finally have sex again with much less pain than before. And I am positive that I can be completely pain free by doing my exercises."

Typical Renew Program For Women™ Routine

Ending Female Pain is best used as a foundation to your self-care and healing journey. Read the whole book before creating your first body-mind routine. By reading all four parts of the book first, you will be better able to integrate the tools and techniques into a life-changing strategy to help you take control of your pain. Remember to be gentle with yourself. If you fall off the horse, don't beat yourself up. Instead, make a decision to transform your condition and to change your outlook towards your condition from sufferer to empowered woman.

What can you expect to feel when you begin your program? You may experience emotional release, muscle soreness, or short-term exacerbation of pain. You may feel some or all of these symptoms before your momentum builds up and you begin to defeat your pain.

Your typical routine should be based on a Monday to Sunday approach. Your program needs to include activities every day of the week to combat and defeat whichever condition or combination of conditions that have led you to read this book. You will have to dedicate at least one hour per day to yourself to overcome your condition. Break up your routine into smaller parts during the course of the day, or set aside a block of time in the evening and complete your whole routine at that time. Incorporate the techniques into your daily life. Stretch at work, meditate over morning coffee, and end your day with your trigger point releases and a warm herbal bath.

Table 2.1: Typical Beginning Daily Routine

SCHEDULE	ACTION ITEM	MORE INFO
Tuesday & Thursday	Foam rolling and Pilates	Part II
Monday-Wednesday-Friday	Yoga stretching series	Part II
Daily	Hands-on self-care techniques	Part III
Daily	Kegels/reverse Kegels	Part II
Daily	Mind/Body visualizations	Part IV
Daily	Keep your mind aware of the PFM toolbox	Part IV

Mind–Body Routine

Although stress does not cause pelvic pain, it can make it worse. The stress, anxiety and emotional upheaval that accompany chronic pelvic pain can rob you of your day-to-day joys and life experiences. For best results, I recommend that you do at least one mind-body relaxation exercise every day. In times of painful flare-ups, it might be necessary to do the mind-body exercises more often and throughout the day.

I incorporate mind-body techniques into the care of my chronic pelvic pain patients as part of their strategy for success. I also encourage them to seek help from a professional who specializes in this area so they have a way to express the emotional pain they have encountered because of their conditions. The hardest thing for my patients to do is to stop the negative catastrophic thinking that accompanies pelvic pain. Many of my patients develop high levels of hyper-vigilance and "body armor" because of their sexual pain. Look to Part IV of this book for simple-to-implement and easy-to-do relaxation and mind-body techniques.

It is extremely important that all women who have chronic pelvic pain be checked out by a pelvic pain specialist to eliminate pathology and disease. It may also be necessary to seek help from a urologist or urogynecologist as many women with chronic pelvic pain also have bladder issues. Many times my patients have to augment the exercises and tools in this book with medications to ease pain, decrease spasms, elevate mood levels, control hormone levels, or deal with bladder issues. Whatever your specific medical needs are, you must have caregivers that specialize in pelvic pain as partners in your health and healing journey.

Pain Mapping/Journaling

Pain mapping is a critical component to your success. Get to know Tables 2.2 and 2.3 on pages 26 and 27 as you begin to map and rate your pain level. Table 2.2 is a basic pain-mapping chart. Use it to map your progress during your intra-vaginal work. For example, chart your pain like this: "My pain is in layer one at 3 o'clock rating at 8/10" (i.e., 0= no pain and 10= worst pain ever). Moving forward, you have an objective measurement to chart your progress. More details on pelvic layers can be found in Chapter 3, page 33.

Table 2.2: Mapping Your Intra-Vaginal Pelvic Pain

PDF version of this table available at http://www.Renew-PT.com

Date	Pelvic Floor Muscle Layer 1, 2, 3	Location of Trigger Point (Use the clock position)	Pain Level 0-10 (0 =no pain, 10 = worst pain)
Ex - 08-02-2009	Ex - Layer 3	Ex - 9 o'clock	7/10 pain, refers to the right labia

Recommendation: Keep a Pain and Progress Diary

Track your routine and progress in a systematic and objective manner. Doing this will let you know which techniques and exercises are working in your healing routine. Your program will evolve, but with the large selection of methods and exercises to choose from, you can mix and match until you get the perfect balance. Any worsening of your symptoms is normal in the beginning until a steady state is reached. You can download the following table at *www.Renew-PT.com* so you can keep a weekly diary of your progress and pain levels.

Table 2.3: Weekly Pain and Progress Diary

PDF version of this table available at http://www.Renew-PT.com

Date	Location of Pain	Pain Level 0-10 (0 =no pain, 10 = worst pain)	Techniques Used for Pain Relief	Emotional States Relaxation Technique Used
Ex - 08-02-09	Ex - Gluteal	Ex - 8/10	Ex - • Exercise • Foam Roller • Massage • Trig. Point	• Unable to relax • Soap bubbles visualization

Let's Get Started

Now that you have a road map, all you have to do is to get started. Begin today. Do not delay. Do not get overwhelmed. Sometimes it's easier to just start off slowly and then add different parts as you go. Start with things that are familiar to you. The more painful your condition, the more you will have to incorporate the techniques, methods and exercises in this book in order to manage your pelvic pain. In the beginning, you should expect to spend at least one hour a day on your "Renew Program For Women™" using the methods and exercises in this book. It is the only way to fight back. Even if you have a busy day and can only spare 5 minutes, it's better than doing nothing at all.

The self-care techniques and exercises in this book will become more familiar and easier to do the more you practice them. What I have given you are many choices. When creating your routine, choose the things that work well for you. Many of my patients become frustrated if they do not get immediate results. Be realistic. If you've had this condition for 6 months to several years, it will take time to get better. Sometimes you will feel as if you are experiencing a setback. This is quite normal as your muscles have not been worked out in this manner before. If you get really sore, cut back and be gentler with the stretches and techniques, or take a day off to rest and let your body recover. You must find the right amount of exercise for your body, your needs and your pain levels. The critical thing is not to give up but to persevere against a condition that is threatening to steal your life away from you. You must be in warrior frame-of-mind, with heart and soul strong, especially in times of painful flare-ups.

Never give up. Do something each day that brings you closer to defeating your pelvic pain. Be the heroine in your own story.

Chapter Three

"The greatest mistake you can make in life is to continually be afraid you will make one."
—Elbert Hubbard

Chapter 3

PELVIC FLOOR MUSCLE CONDITIONS: BACKGROUND

Before we get into the techniques, exercises and strategies for ending female pain, it is important to first understand your body on an anatomical level, a physiological level, and an energy level. Your pelvic floor is a complex set of muscles, nerves, and connective tissues like fascia that can accurately be called the cradle or basket of your being. On an energy level, the pelvic floor contains the first chakra, or energy center, and more importantly, supports the other chakras. So if the foundation is experiencing stress and trauma, then naturally all of your energy will be affected. Major nerves that innervate your entire lower extremity pass through the pelvic area, and a complex web of muscles support your vagina, bladder, uterus, intestines, and other abdominal organs. If the muscles in your pelvic floor are in spasm, or are filled with trigger points, your pain can be both excruciating and debilitating.

To understand this area of your body better, we'll take a look at the various constructs of your pelvic floor muscles, also called the levator ani muscles. We will also define conditions like vulvodynia, dyspareunia, vaginismus, and scar adhesions, and explore states of the muscle tissue like trigger points and muscle spasms. There is a lot to cover here and throughout the book, so remember to consult the extensive glossary as well to familiarize yourself with key concepts and terms found in this book.

I have also included in this chapter the basics of conducting your own visual and topical vaginal exam. You have to embrace your vagina. This may sound strange, but many of my patients are afraid to look at their vaginas which they consider ugly, or are disconnected with their pelvic floor muscles. Let me tell you straight out – your vagina is a wonderful area of your body to explore and get to know. Do not be ashamed of it. By getting to know your own anatomy and its particular nuances, you will find that you can open the door to your own healing and evolve your condition to a state of reduced pain, and more importantly, maintain long-term results. You hold the key to getting on the road to recovery.

Understanding How Your Pelvic Floor Muscles Work
Diagram 3.1: Pelvic Floor Muscles – 3rd Layer

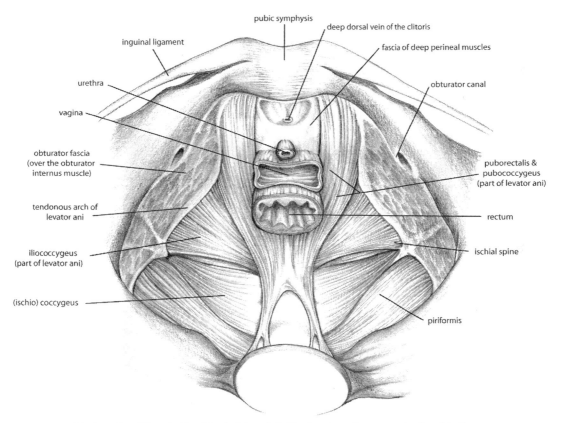

Top down view of the pelvic floor. Your body is cut in half at the waist and you are peering down into the 3rd layer of the pelvic floor basket with organs removed. Illustration by Winston Johnson

The overall pelvic floor muscle group has three primary functions. First, they are supportive and hold your organs up. Second, they are sphinctoric and help prevent urinary and fecal incontinence. Third, they are sexual, enhancing and making orgasms stronger and better. The pelvic

Diagram 3.2: Pelvic Floor Muscles - 1st and 2nd Layer

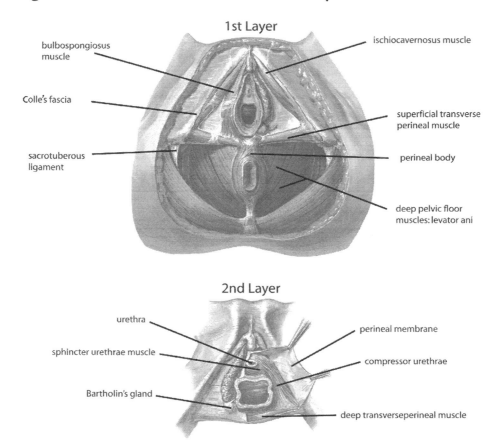

The second layer muscles appear in the diagram below the first and are found behind the Layer 1 muscles listed on the top of this diagram. Source - Netter Images

floor muscles are innervated by the pudendal nerve, perineal nerve, inferior rectal nerve, the sacral spinal and levator ani nerves. These nerves originate in the low back and tailbone region anatomically known as the L4-S4 region.

The muscles of the female pelvic floor can be a source of confusion for many people – even to the trained professional – because they have been given several different names, making it difficult to understand the nomenclature and classification. In this book we will classify the female pelvic muscles into three layers and will describe other structures that are necessary to understand in order to perform the techniques described in Part III of this book. Please look at

Table 3.1 on page 34 for a description of the main muscles and anatomy of the female pelvic floor. Use the accompanying anatomy Diagrams 3.1, 3.2 and 3.3 to refer back as you begin to absorb and understand the techniques I have compiled for pelvic pain relief. Be scientific in your approach to better visualize the musculature of your own body.

The pelvic floor muscles themselves are divided into three layers, with each layer progressively deeper inside the vagina or rectum. Using your index finger as a road map, the first layer corresponds to the first knuckle, the second layer corresponds to the second knuckle and the deeper layer corresponds to the third knuckle. Now let's think about the vaginal opening looking like a clock (see Diagram 3.3). Twelve o'clock is by the clitoris, six o'clock by the rectum, three o'clock to the left side and nine o'clock to the right. Now imagine that each layer is also its own clock. So you have three clocks, one at each level,

Diagram 3.3: Pelvic Floor Muscles Layer by Layer

The three pelvic floor muscle layers, each corresponding to a knuckle of the index finger. The inset shows the clock concept of the 1st layer. Think of each layer as having its own clock as you begin to map and track your pain.
Source for base images: Netter Images

which is how I want you to visualize the pelvic floor muscles as you begin to digest the techniques in Part III. Thinking this way will help you locate problematic areas of your pelvic floor muscles, and will help you track your progress as you begin to understand and unravel the sources of your pain.

Table 3.1: Anatomy of Pelvic Floor Muscle Layers

LAYER NAME	MAIN MUSCLES	MAIN STRUCTURES IN LAYER
- Layer 1 - Located first knuckle of the index finger - Also called Urogenital triangle	- Superficial transverse perineal muscle - Ischiocavernosus - Bulbocavernosus - External Genitalia: includes urethra, lower vagina, vulva, mons pubis, labia majora, labia minora, clitoris, vestibular bulb, Bartholin's glands	- Colle's fascia - Vaginal/urethral openings - External female genitalia - Pubic symphysis and pubic ramibones
- Layer 2 - Located second knuckle of the index finger - Also called Urogenital diaphragm	- Sphincter urethrae - Deep transverse perineal muscle - Compressor urethrae muscle	- Bartholin's glands - Urethra - Perineal membrane - Vagina
- Layer 3 - Located third knuckle of the index finger - Also called Pelvic diaphragm	- Levator ani: Commonly broken down into pubococcygeus, puborectalis, iliococcygeus - Obturator internus - Ischicoccygeus (coccygeus)	- Tendinous arch of levator ani muscle - Obturator fascia - Sacrotuberous & sacrospinous ligament

Definitions of Muscle States –
Finding Your Trigger Points Is the First Step to Healing

Trigger points are one of the most important concepts to understand as you begin to dissect your pain. Loosely defined, trigger points are a section of muscle tissue that is stuck in its contracted state. Trigger points are knot-like spots – the most well-known example being the ones we sometimes get in our necks and trapezius muscle that create a burning and stabbing pain. Trigger points in the pelvic floor are quite similar to the ones we all get in these.

On a more anatomical and physiological level, trigger points are taut muscular bands that are the result of an injury to the motor end plate of the muscle cells. Trigger points in the pelvic floor muscles can be activated by stress, visceral or organ pain, pelvic and hip malalignment, chronic pelvic floor muscle holding, hormonal imbalances, prolonged sitting or pressure on the pelvic muscles.

Dr. Janet Travell and Dr. David Simons, pioneering experts in trigger point therapy, categorize trigger points as latent and active. The latent trigger points don't actively refer pain but cause pain when touched. Active trigger points can refer pain to another muscle or body part without actually being touched. Once trigger points are present or latent, they can become especially active with stress, strain, and injury to the muscle.

Specifically in the pelvic floor muscles, or PFMs, trigger points can elicit pain when touched or cause other symptoms like urinary urgency and frequency, feelings

Diagram 3.4: Effects of Trigger Points on Sarcomeres

Normal muscle fibers with equidistant sarcomeres (muscle cells).
2- Trigger point shows contracted muscle fibers with outer muscle bands stretched out.

of pain with sitting, low back pain, sacroiliac (SI joint) pain, abdominal or hip pain, rectal discomfort, and pain with intercourse. Most of the trigger point techniques found in Part III will help locate and get rid of active or latent trigger points in the pelvic floor muscles, ones that when pressed cause a tremendous amount of pain or refer pain to an associated body part. Finding external trigger points that refer pain to the pelvic floor is a more difficult task, and I recommend that you work with a physical therapist that specializes in pelvic floor muscle therapy to help you make the connections to the root referral trigger point. For example, many of my patients have active trigger points in their lower backs around vertebrae L5, S1, S2 that refer pain into their pelvic floor muscles. Once located, I am able to incorporate self-healing techniques into my patients' programs, but you will need your physical therapist to do some of the detective work to unravel this part of your pain.

In conclusion, it is imperative that you begin to understand how the trigger point mechanism is at work in your own body. Once you find your trigger points, use the techniques in this book to help eliminate pain and to help reeducate the pelvic floor muscles so they have less tension, more flexibility, more range of motion, and almost always, less pain.

"The Pain Down There"

My patients want to know what caused their "pain down there." For many, their pelvic pain started acutely and then developed into a chronic condition afflicting them for months and sometimes years. Many of the women I treat tell me that their vulvar pain developed after an infection, surgical procedure, traumatic fall, or as a result of giving birth. One common thread is the devastating effects their pain has had on their lives and oftentimes on their relationships.

In my healing center, my patients report symptoms like painful sex, inability to sit for more than 10 minutes or to walk without pain, and discomfort in wearing certain clothes such as jeans, panty hose or thong underwear. Many of them suffer from sexual dysfunction or are depressed because their pain has taken their sex lives away from them. Although most of my patients are in their 20s and 30s, I also see older women suffering from these conditions as well. These women describe their pain as tingling, burning, or knife-like. Their vaginas feel raw and itchy. These symptoms can be constant or intermittent, and their pain can rate from low level to incapacitating.

Other complaints I hear from patients are clitoral pain, labial pain, groin pain, low back pain, pain in their sit bones, pain with defecation, and increased pain during their menstrual cycle. Many report vaginal dryness and redness and skin irritation that can extend to their inner thigh muscles. Others have cuts and sores in their vaginas. Some feel heaviness in their pelvis, as if there is something falling out of their vaginas. Many also describe episodes of extreme pain with penetration, called dyspareunia, and for many, this pain can linger for hours or days after their sexual encounter is over. Many tell me they have lingering pain after orgasms. One of my patients reported such intense pain after an orgasm that it made her double over in pain and cry. I have been compiling symptoms as reported by my patients for several years in an effort to discern patterns. In Table 3.2, I have created a symptoms table for you to use as a single reference to gain insight and understanding into what you are reporting as "the pain down there."

Table 3.2: Typical Symptoms of "The Pain Down There"

ORIGINS OF SYMPTOMS	SYMPTOMS AS REPORTED BY MY PATIENTS
Emotional (usually in combination with other symptoms)	- Catastrophic thinking - Isolation - Strained relationships with partners - Depression - Sadness - Guilt - Sleep disturbances - Suicidal tendencies/thoughts - Emotionally unavailable
Muscular	- Pain in the gluteal or back muscles, knees, or abdominal area - Generalized soreness in PFM muscles - PFM spasms - PFM trigger points - Constant or sharp-like pains in muscles associated or near the vagina - Pelvic floor muscle weakness
Rectal	- Bleeding with defecation - Constipation - Pain with defecation - Redness around the anus - Burning-like pain - Itching - Pushing to get feces out - Feelings of pelvic pressure - Pain in the rectum after orgasms - Pain or irritation with thong underwear
Skin	-Allergies to metals, perfumes - Sensitive skin - Irritation with certain toilet papers, tampons or sanitary napkins - Itching - Sensitivity to soaps - Painful scars - Feelings of vaginal swelling - Burning pain in the labia - Constant ache throughout the vulva - Raw feeling in the vaginal tissues

ORIGINS OF SYMPTOMS	SYMPTOMS AS REPORTED BY MY PATIENTS
Vaginal	- Painful intercourse - Vaginal itching, burning, rawness - Constant awareness of vaginal area with certain clothing - Pain with touching/wiping - Pain at opening or deep inside - Clitoral pain - Labial pain - Cuts in the vagina - Skin patches of varying colors - Pelvic pressure – feels like something is falling out of the vagina
Urinary	- Painful urination - Urgency and frequency of urination - Suprapubic pain - Hesitancy in getting urine out - Slow urine stream - Feelings of incomplete emptying - Habit of pushing urine out - Vaginal stinging with urination - Urethral pain - Feelings of pelvic pressure - Leaking with coughing, sneezing or laughing

If you have any of the symptoms I have described in Table 3.2, you might be suffering from one of the many conditions that affect the pelvic floor area. What are the most common conditions called? Most cases fall under the umbrella of vulvodynia, vestibulodynia, dyspareunia, vaginismus, interstitial cystitis, pudendal nerve entrapment, pelvic floor muscle spasm or dysfunction, lichen schlerosis, endometriosis/fibroids, and scar pain. Let's take a moment to examine each of these conditions. It is important to note that most of my patients have some combination of conditions that are contributing to their overall pain. As you take a look at each condition, you may very well discover that your symptoms point towards multiple contributing factors. Don't worry. First and foremost, we need to separate and identify each factor that is causing your pain so that you can devise the best approach to attacking and ultimately defeating the pain that is controlling your life right now.

Table 3.3: Leading Theories on the Causes of "The Pain Down There"

What Is Thought to Cause "The Pain Down There"? (Usually a Combination)
- Antibiotics
- Autoimmune disorders
- Back injuries
- Bacterial vaginosis
- Bladder problems, such as interstitial cystitis
- Candidiasis
- Childbirth causing trauma to the pelvic floor structures
- Chronic yeast infections
- Chronic infections relating to pelvic, hip muscles and abdominal organs
- Cesarean section
- Damage to nerves that innervate the pelvic area/organs or hypersensitive nerves that innervate the pelvic area
- Damage to sensory nerves of the pelvic area
- Endometriosis
- Episiotomy, perineal tearing
- Falling on coccyx or tailbone
- Fibroids
- Genital herpes
- Herniated disc
- Hip replacement surgeries and hip labral tears
- High oxalates in urine
- Hormonal problems
- Injury to the nerves that innervate the vulva
- Interstitial cystitis
- Lumbar disc problems
- Neuropathy
- Organ prolapse-bladder, uterus, or rectum
- Pelvic floor muscle spasms and trigger points
- Prolonged use of birth control pills
- Pudenal nerve damage or entrapment
- Referred pain from areas adjacent to the pelvic floor
- Repetitive stress injuries affecting the pelvis
- Sacrum injuries/surgeries

What Is Thought to Cause "The Pain Down There"? (Usually a Combination)
- Sexual abuse/rape
- Spinal fusions of the lumbar spine
- Sports injuries such as bike riding
- Straining with defecation and urination
- Surgical procedures to the pelvic/abdominal area and resulting scar adhesions
- Trauma to the pelvic area
- Trauma, injury, traction or entrapment of the pudenal nerve
- Trichomonas infections
- Vaginal atrophy secondary in menopause due to lack of estrogen
- Vulvar dermatosis

The definitive and concrete causes of all pelvic floor disorders have eluded medical professionals. What I have done here is to compile a list of the leading theories. Again, most of my patients report several causes that have contributed to their conditions.

Medical Conditions Affecting the Pelvic Floor Muscles
Vulvodynia

Vulvodynia is an umbrella term used to describe pelvic pain. There are actually several variations among which it is important to draw a distinction. Many of my patients have difficulty pinpointing their vulvar pain. They say it hurts "everywhere down there," which is called generalized vulvodynia. For others, the pain is at specific spots in their vulvas such as in their vestibules, which is called localized vulvodynia or sometimes called vestibulodynia. For some, their pain is worse during and right before their periods, or pain comes on all of a sudden, which is called unprovoked vulvodynia. Pain is sometimes also felt with direct contact to the vagina such as when wiping or with sexual intercourse. This is called provoked vulvodynia. Many also report they cannot have any penetration because the penis cannot get in the vagina (vaginismus).

The causes for vulvodynia are largely unknown and are thought to be multi-faceted. There is no evidence that vulvodynia is caused directly by sexually transmitted diseases or infections. Recent research has put a lot of emphasis on the nerves that innervate the pelvic and vaginal area, indicating that vulvodynia is a result of a neuropathic condition where the nerves are not functioning properly. Table 3.3 lists many of the possible causes of vulvodynia. Whatever the root cause, many gynecologists, urologists and caregivers agree that the pelvic floor muscles are deeply affected, and many times normalizing their function can bring great relief to pelvic pain sufferers.

Childbirth

Childbirth is a major culprit of sexual pain and pelvic floor muscle dysfunction in women. The pelvic floor muscles are stretched to their limits during delivery and the pelvic nerves also undergo traction and stretching, often compromising their function. While these are all natural occurrences during birth, once coupled with perineal tears, episiotomies, C-sections, and assisted deliveries using vacuums and forceps, the birth trauma can be quickly compounded.

In obstetrics and gynecology pelvic trauma during birth is classified into degrees of tears. A first-degree tear is classified as a tear through vaginal mucosa and perineal skin only, a second degree tear is a tear that extends into the perineal muscles, a third degree tear involves a tear that extends into the external sphincter, and a fourth degree tear is a laceration affecting the anal sphincter and anal rectal mucosa. No matter what the level of the tear it is the opinion of this author that women should be routinely referred to a pelvic floor specialist after birth, and most definitely uro-gynecological rehabilitation should be prescribed routinely to all women after pelvic surgeries. In many other countries, such as France, pelvic rehab is routinely prescribed to new moms, but in the US this is not the common practice.

New moms come to me with varying complaints including pain with sitting while breastfeeding, pain with sexual intercourse, urinary leaking, fecal incontinence, perineal scar pain or C-section pain. To facilitate recovery after child-birth, I emphasize pre-natal pelvic education to solidify strategies for success. For example, pregnant women need to be empowered with information and made aware that cetain positions are less likely to cause perineal tearing.

They also need to know that perineal massage started religiously at 34 weeks of pregnancy is a great preparation for labor and helps prepare the PFMs for the upcoming stretching during labor. It is also very important for pregnant women to choose a healthcare provider who will not routinely perform episiotomies unless absolutely necessary.

Vestibulodynia

Vestibulodynia is a localized, provoked form of vulvodynia, in which particu-lar areas of the vestibule show certain characteristics. The vestibule is the oval shaped area around the opening of the vagina. This condition, sometimes also called vulvar vestibulitis is one of the most common sexual pains I treat. Vestibu-lodynia is characterized by three criteria that were first proposed by researcher Friedrich EG. Jr. in 1987, in the *Journal of Reproductive Medicine, 32:110-114*. The 3 main characteristics as described by Friedrich are:

1. Pain when the vestibule is palpated with a cotton swab. This is called the "Q-tip test" and is described in greater detail in this chapter in the section on vaginal self-examination.

2. Erythema, or redness throughout the vestibule that can sometimes extend to the labia majora and inner thighs.

3. Severe pain with vaginal penetration of the penis, speculum, tampon, finger, or dilator.

The pain felt in the vestibule is thought to be caused by a proliferation of intraepithelial nerve endings found in the vestibular mucosa. Research also shows that these nerve endings contain a compound called calcium gene related peptide. This compound is found in C-fiber nerves which are present in the vestibule. The research indicates that women with vestibulodynia have 10 times more C-fiber pain nerves in the vestibules than normal women. It is thought that this increase in C-fiber nerve endings is one of the major culprits contributing to the excruciating pain felt by women suffering from this condition.

Another possible culprit is the hyperactivity of mast cells in the vestibule. These cells play a part in the inflammatory process and also produce, among other compounds, nerve growth factor which is thought to help turn normal nerves that process pain signals into neuropathic nerves that produce pain signals no matter what the external stimulus may be.

Pudendal Nerve Entrapment

As the pudendal nerve travels on its journey from the lower back nerve root through the pelvis, the pudendal nerve can easily become entrapped and squeezed by fascia, muscles, and ligaments. Furthermore, a woman's pudendal nerve can become injured during childbirth, excessive bike riding, falls, accidents, etc., and once the nerve becomes entrapped or injured it can create horrific, deep and agonizing pain that refers directly to the pelvic floor. An injured pudendal nerve can cause pain with sitting, pain in the labia, or pain in the clitoris. Some of my patients with pudendal nerve entrapment have even reported a feeling like their pubic hair is being pulled or yanked out. To resolve this condition, you need to work with a team that includes a physical therapist with pelvic floor specialty and a urogynecologist or urologist who specializes in pudendal nerve neuralgias. Typically, the medical doctor might inject the area to calm down the pain, and then you would come to see me and I would get to work to reduce the muscle spasms and release the nerve. Many times, but only as a last resort, surgery is the only option for many women suffering from pudendal nerve entrapment.

Vaginismus

Vaginismus occurs when the muscles of the pelvic floor go into involuntary contraction, creating spasms that close the vaginal opening. Patients with vaginismus find it difficult, if not impossible, to have sex because of these severe spasms in the outer layer of the vagina. Pain in the hips, lower back, and gluteal muscles is reported as well, which makes daily activities challenging. These patients have sexual desire but the contracted muscles do not allow the penis to enter into the vagina without pain. Vaginismus is best treated with manual stretching of the pelvic floor muscles and with medical dilators as described in Part III. With proper self-care, the affected muscles release their spasms and trigger points and become softer and more supple, making sexual penetration possible.

Fibromyalgia

Fibromyalgia syndrome affects the muscles, tendons, ligaments, and soft tissues of the body. Patients generally complain of pain throughout the entire body, including the vulvar and pelvic/hip region. Additional symptoms include extreme fatigue, sleep disturbances, and burning sensations throughout the body. Fibromyalgia sufferers have multiple trigger points and tender spots all over their bodies that when pressed elicit pain. To diagnose fibromyalgia, a good physician relies on a detailed medical history, and checks for pain and tenderness in 11 out of 18 specified trigger point areas along with locating painful areas in the body that have persisted for more than three months. For more detailed information about fibromyalgia visit a great online resource called *www.FMaware.org*.

Interstitial Cystitis

Interstitial cystitis, or IC, is a medical condition that produces pain in the bladder and urethra. IC is also known as painful bladder syndrome, and patients with IC often report symptoms of pain in the vulva, pain with intercourse, and pain in the lower back and hips. Other common complaints include urinary urgency – a feeling of an urgent need to urinate, or urinary frequency. Sometimes, the frequency can be extreme. I have had patients who go to the bathroom every 5 to10 minutes. Another common symptom is pain when the bladder is full, and patients often report that the pain subsides after urination. I recommend my IC patients keep a food diary, as there are many bladder irritants that can lead to painful flare-ups and contribute to excruciating pain if consumed. Here is a list of foods to avoid if you have been diagnosed with IC:

1. Fruit juices such as orange, cranberry, tomato, or lemon juice are bladder irritants.

2. Caffeine stimulates bladder nerves, causing pain, inflammation, and irritation to the bladder. Increased bladder nerve stimulation will also produce an increase in urinary frequency.

3. Regular or green teas because of the tannic acid found in them.

4. Regular and diet sodas because of citric acid, artificial flavoring, preservatives, and carbonation.

5. Artificial sweeteners are thought to be bladder irritants.

6. Chocolate and cocoa products may irritate the bladder lining.

7. Wine and alcohol are potential bladder irritants.

For more information on IC, visit Jill Osborne's amazing web portal at *www.IC-Network.com*. She has done a great job of providing all of the latest information.

Dyspareunia

Dyspareunia is a general term that refers to painful intercourse. This pain can occur before, during, or after sexual activity. There are many causes of dyspareunia including atrophic vaginitis, vulvar vestibulitis, lichen schlerosis, endometriosis, scar adhesions, and psychological trauma such as sexual abuse.

Endometriosis

I treat many women who experience sexual pain as a result of endometriosis. The uterus is lined with a specific tissue called endometrial epithelium stroma. When this tissue grows outside of the uterus it is called endometriosis. This condition can cause a lot of pain and many other problems in a woman's body. Endometrial tissue can be found anywhere in the pelvis, such as the ovaries, uterus, fallopian tubes, intestines, bladder and colon. Most women with endometriosis usually experience pelvic pains during their menstrual cycles, but many also have excruciating pain that is not related to their periods. Endometriosis can cause not only sexual pain but also infertility, as the tissue growths can affect fallopian tubes, ovaries and the proper functioning of the uterus. If adhesions and scar tissue related to endometriosis build up, it can lead to a condition called frozen pelvis. If you think you are suffering from endometriosis you must make sure you are comfortable with your caregivers. Find one who always works closely with a gynecologist that specializes in endometriosis, as surgery is often performed in conjunction with physical therapy to achieve results.

Adhesions/Scar Pain

Post-surgical scar adhesions occur in women after most pelvic and abdominal surgeries. An adhesion is a fibrous band of scar tissue that forms between internal organs and tissues, joining them together abnormally. Adhesions form after surgery as part of the normal healing process and help to limit the spread of infection. Sometimes though, adhesions cause tissues to grow together that normally would not be connected. Millions of people worldwide suffer from painful adhesions after surgery, and data has suggested over 50 percent of women will develop scar adhesions following gynecologic and non-gynecological surgeries (*Obmanagement.com, June 2003, Vol. 15, No. 6*). In my experience, the longer a woman waits to seek therapy for her scars, the denser and tougher the scar adhesions become. More importantly, scar adhesions may be associated with pelvic pain and sexual pain, abnormalities of bowel function, and infertility.

I have seen many women develop overall pelvic pain because of adhesions after surgical procedures such as C-sections, myomectomy, hysterectomy, laparoscopic procedures, episiotomy, vestibulectomy, hymenectomy, perineal tearing, and even vulvar biopsies.

How to Perform a Self-Examination of the Vulva-Vaginal Area

Now that you have a basic understanding of the symptoms, general causes and various conditions that can afflict pelvic floor muscles and tissues, it is important to take the time to get to know your own body. You cannot be successful with your own self-care unless you take the time to examine yourself and learn to understand the uniqueness of your body. Many of the women I treat start out in my healing center completely disconnected to their pelvic floor muscles and vaginas. I tell them that they have to change this outlook in order to have any chance of success. Get to know your body first so you can get on the road to recovery and long-term results.

Make sure to perform your exam in a well-lit place. If the area you are in is poorly lit, you will need additional lighting. You will also need a mirror, Q-tip and lubricant.

There are many positions in which you can perform your vulva examination. It is important to find a position that you are comfortable in and allows you to examine the whole area. Recommended positions for this examination are sitting with legs apart or standing with one leg up or squatting over a mirror.

Hold your mirror up close to examine all the external parts. To examine the inner parts you will have to spread your vaginal lips to expose the vulvar area.

Checking All the Parts

The vulva is made up of the following structures: labia majora, labia minora, clitoris, vestibule of the vagina, bulb of the vestibule, and the glands of Bartholin. We will also be examining the perineum in addition to the vulva.

Diagram 3.5: External Genitalia, Part of Layer 1 of the Pelvic Floor Muscles

mons pubis

anterior commissure of the labia majora

prepuce of the clitoris

glans of clitoris

external urethral orifice

labia minora

Skene's ducts

labia majora

vestibule of the vagina

Hart's line

hymenal caruncle

vaginal orifice

perineal raphé (cover perineal body)

opening of Bartholin's Glands

anus

Base image: Netter Images

Check Your Mons Pubis

This is the area where your pubic hair and pubic bone are located. Sometimes this is an area of pain for some women who have bladder conditions.

What to Look For

Run your fingers along the skin and feel for any bumps, warts, or sores.

Also examine the area for any color changes in the skin such as red, white or dark spots.

Check Your Clitoris

Feel and look at your clitoris and the surrounding area. Also gently pull back on the hood of the clitoris.

What to Look For

Does the clitoral hood move or is it bound down? The clitoris should freely move in its hood. Also examine the clitoris for coloring, pain and inflammation by lightly touching over it with your finger or Q-tip.

Check Your Labia Minora

These are the inner lips to the right and left of the vaginal opening.

What to Look For

Look and touch by holding the labial skin between thumb and fingers. Check on all sides of the labias – front and back and both sides right and left. Run your fingers along the skin and feel for any bumps, warts, or sores. Examine the area for any color changes in the skin such as red, white or dark spots. Look for ulcers, sores, small blisters, and areas of pain, swelling and inflammation. This area can appear very red and inflamed in women with pelvic floor dysfunction and in women suffering from vulvar vestibulitis.

Check Your Labia Majora

These are your outer vaginal lips next to the labia minora. Slide your fingers along the outer lips both sides. Many of my patients have labial pain, trigger points or itching along the length of the outer labias. Massage and cross friction massage, covered in Part III, work great in reducing pain in this area.

What to Look For

Perform the same examination as for the labia minora.

Check Your Perineum

Although the perineum and the vestibule, the area that surrounds your vaginal opening, are typically not included in the vulva self-examination, I highly recommend that you do not overlook them in your monthly self-care examination. Examining these areas will give you tremendous insight into your pelvic pain condition.

The perineum is the area between your vagina and anus. This is where doctors perform an episiotomy, which is a surgical cut of the perineum done just before the delivery of a child. Many women who experience pain have scar tissue in this area as a result of the episiotomy. This area is a highway for many muscles and it provides us with an external view of the levator ani muscles, also known as pelvic floor muscles. Palpation or touching of this area will give you an idea about what is going on internally in your pelvic floor muscles such as mobility and pain.

What to Look For

First, look for scar tissue, lesions, and sores. Also examine the area for any color changes in the skin such as red, white or dark spots. Many times this area becomes red and hyper-irritable due to the dysfunction that is present in the pelvic floor muscles. When the muscles of the vagina function better, the redness and irritation in this area disappears. You will need a mirror and to be in a well-lit room for this exam as well.

Now look at the perineal body. This is the midpoint of the perineum. Testing this area for mobility and ease of movement will give you an insight to what is going on in your pelvic muscles. When performing your pelvic drops, pelvic floor muscle release, or reverse Kegels, this is the area you want to see drop down, release or come forward towards your mirror. Many times I will instruct my patients to gently move this area to the left, right, up, and down and to feel which direction it is not moving freely. Once you have established that, stretch the perineal body into that direction by holding it in the stretch position for 30 seconds to one minute. I cover this in greater detail in Part III.

Q-tip Test

The Q-tip test is an essential method for determining the levels of inflammation and pain in the vestibule. As you progress on your healing journey, you will continually perform the Q-tip test and track your results. In ideal settings the Q-tip test should elicit no pain. If you experience any pain with this test, consult a physician or physical therapist that specializes in pelvic pain immediately.

Diagram 3.6: Location of Hart's Line

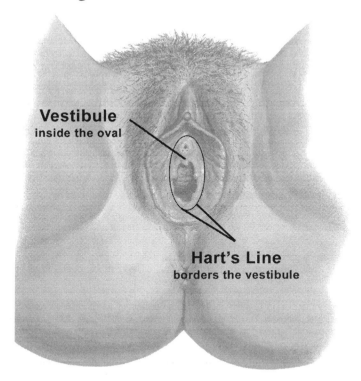

Perform the Q-tip test along Hart's Line
Base images: Netter Images

Where is the vestibule? The vulvar vestibule forms an oval shape around the opening of the vagina. The top is bordered by the clitoris, the bottom by the posterior fourchette, the inner sides by the hymenal remnants and the outer parts of the oval by the labia minora. Additional structures found in the vulvar vestibule include the major and minor vestibular glands, Skene's Gland and the urethra.

To perform this test you will need a mirror and a Q-tip with a small amount of lubricant. Locate the line that separates the labia minora from the vestibule. This is called Hart's Line. Once you locate it with your mirror, imagine the vestibule as a clock, with the clitoris at twelve o'clock, the left at three o'clock, the anus at six o'clock, and the right at nine o'clock. Using very gentle pressure, go around the clock from one o'clock to twelve o'clock. As you perform this test, rate the level of pain you experience from 0 to 10 (i.e., 0 = no pain, 5 = moderate pain, 10 = worst pain ever). If this test elicits any pain you probably have some form of vestibulodynia. Make sure to keep track of your painful areas with your Q-tip.

Vaginal Scars

During your examination, you may come across old scars that you may not have noticed before. Scars and tears in the perineum can often be a source of sexual pain. Vaginal scars are frequently the result of episiotomies or tearing during childbirth, or surgical procedures such as biopsies and vestibulodectomies. It is possible for the perineum to tear during childbirth or sexual activity. Check out your scars for proper healing, pain and mobility. If the scar feels thick, is painful or has a discharge, have it checked by your gynecologist. If the scar is raised, painful, thick or feels tight, there are ways to reduce pain, stretch the scar, and restore motion to the tissues. Trigger points may exist in these perineal scars and refer pain to the vulva and pelvic floor muscles. See Part III of this book for treatment and healing techniques for perineum scars.

Diagram 3.7: Clock Concept for Hart's Line Test

Base image: Netter Images

We've just covered the basics of your pelvic floor muscles and structures, both internally and externally. Remember you must get to know your own anatomy, with its nuances and uniqueness. Now let's get ready in this next section of the book where we will build our foundation, with Kegels, ball strengthening, yoga stretching, at-work strategies, and foam rolling.

Part 2
Exercises and Stretches for the Relief of Pelvic Pain

"We are what we repeatedly do.
Excellence, therefore,
is not an act but a habit."
— Aristotle

Chapter 4

TO KEGEL OR NOT TO KEGEL

The term *Kegel*, developed by gynecologist Dr. Arnold Kegel, is used to describe a set of exercises that is designed to improve the function of the pelvic floor muscles. The problem is that there are subtle nuances to Kegels that if not taken into account, can actually produce worse results for patients with pelvic pain. Typically, basic Kegels are prescribed for women suffering from incontinence or organ prolapse, and are designed to help strengthen the PFMs, improve coordination, continence and sexual function by reducing laxity and decreasing weakness.

When I evaluate a typical woman suffering from pelvic pain, I frequently find that in addition to muscle weakness, the PFMs usually have excessive tone, increased shortness, extreme tension, spasms and multiple trigger points in them, rather than laxity. I also often find a lack of flexibility in the muscles that attach to the pelvis such as the inner thighs, hip flexors, gluteal and abdominal muscles. The PFMs are normally in a relaxed state, and they respond to what is happening in your body and mind. They can respond to thoughts, past experiences, trauma, visceral problems, abnormal breathing patterns and pain. Usually, their response to any of the above is to become tense. This tension can go on for years, resulting in shortened muscle fibers filled with spasms, trigger points, and myofascial restrictions.

Once the muscle fibers get shorter and tenser, they are typically weaker. The weakness is not due to looseness, as in the typical incontinence or prolapse patient. Instead, the weakness is caused by muscles which are too tight or hypertonic. The shortened muscle has the ability to contract, but the contractions are weak because there is a decrease in the fiber's ability to move. This type of weakness leads to urinary leaking and urge and frequency of urination, which are typical complaints I hear from my patients with pelvic pain. To effectively treat these hypertonic muscle fibers, they first need to be lengthened and relaxed before they can be strengthened and toned. So the prescription of regular Kegels, where you are told simply to draw up your muscles to prevent leaking or pain, does not work. In fact it can lead to more pain and weakness as muscle fibers become even shorter, and more hypertonic. As a result, the PFMs often develop more trigger points in them.

In order to accomplish the release, I recommend that my patients do a daily, reverse Kegel release program first and then embark on a Kegel strengthening program for their muscles once they master the muscle relaxation and release techniques. Having first lengthened the muscles, the fibers can then be better strengthened, leading to reduced pain, improved continence, and enhanced sexual response.

The Kegel programs I have created are to be performed on several levels, beginning with the reverse Kegels to relax the muscles, followed by strengthening with the contract, relax, and the quick-flicks kegels once you have mastered the reverse series. This order is necessary because the release is needed first before you can strengthen both slow twitch and fast twitch fibers of the PFMs. By understanding some of the nuances of the types of Kegels. I will describe in the following paragraphs, you can achieve better success and gain better control over your pain.

Reverse Kegel Muscle Relaxation Series

Your ability to have conscious release of the pelvic floor muscles is a critical part of your recovery program. The foundation of conscious and mindful release is the mastering of the reverse Kegel relaxation exercises. Your success in all of the other techniques in Part III of this book rests on the reverse Kegel series I describe in this chapter. You must learn to focus on and relax these muscles before they can become functional again and pain-free. Relaxation and lengthening of the PFMs with reverse Kegels is also called downtraining. To ensure success with your overall program, you need to do reverse Kegels and downtraining along with the techniques in Part III of this book, which include PFM massage, trigger point, pressure, and myofascial release as well as intra-vaginal dilator stretching.

The reverse Kegel downtraining series contains eight techniques that will help you gain awareness and control over your pelvic floor. In the beginning, work hard to master the release techniques, and then you can incorporate this focus while performing the other sexual healing tools throughout this book. It is extremely important that you practice your relaxation exercises throughout the day. Do not go through an 8-hour work day without releasing the tension in your muscles. The following exercises are easy to perform and can be done anywhere or anytime. At first the PFM relaxation exercises will be extremely difficult to visualize and perform. Many of you have had tension and pain in these muscles for a very long time. Like anything else, the more you practice these exercises, the easier they will become to do and to implement. The reverse Kegel series in this book contains the most effective methods that have brought success to my patients. Designed to help you release the tension and then strengthen the PFMs, they are to be used on a daily basis, and especially during flare-ups when they could be used every hour until the pain subsides.

The Importance of Breath

To more effectively perform the reverse Kegel series, you must couple the techniques with proper breathing. When I teach my patients the basics of downtraining, I emphasize diaphragmatic breathing to ensure their success. Diaphragmatic breathing can be defined as a type of breathing that involves the abdominal muscles instead of the ribs, shoulders, and neck muscles. To practice diaphragmatic breathing, place your hand over your belly button. On inhale, let your belly gently rise out into your hands, and on exhale, let the belly flatten. Don't let the breath raise your shoulders, and don't bring your belly in on the inhale and out on the exhale, as this is not diaphragmatic breathing.

The best way to consciously release tension from the PFMs is to try to release the muscles while you inhale. Do not be discouraged if you find this difficult to perform. All of my patients have trouble with this concept in the beginning. Just imagine though, that when you inhale properly, your diaphragm actually lowers to make room for the air, so it is natural to also lower and relax the pelvic floor muscles. When you exhale, your diaphragm rises to push the air out, and you can then raise or contract your PFMs.

It is also important to time your inhalation and exhalation so that they occur over the same length of time. For example, inhale for five seconds, and then exhale for five seconds. I usually recommend to my patients that they inhale for a count of five while consciously dropping and relaxing their PFMs downward. This release and letting go is the hardest exercise to do because many women are not even aware of the tension with which they are holding their PFMs. Once the tension is released, the muscle fibers begin to lengthen. Soon you will be able to release on demand, at which point you can begin a regular Kegel strengthening and toning program.

If you have difficulty coordinating the in-breath with the release, don't let that stop you. It's perfectly alright to do a reverse Kegel with exhalation at first until you master the correct techniques. The most important thing is to increase your awareness and focus and to practice reverse Kegels on a daily basis, even an hourly basis, if needed.

Test Your Progress

Table 4.1: The Renew Physical Therapy Reverse Kegel Self-Grading System

PROGRESS LEVEL	CURRENT CONDITION	ACTION TO BE TAKEN
Level 1	Not able to release PFM	Continue with PFM Release Exercises
Level 2	Able to release PFM a little	Continue with PFM Release Exercises
Level 3	Able to release PFM but not all the way and with some pain	Continue with PFM Release Exercises
Level 4	Able to release PFM completely without pain or with some pain	Start Kegel Strengthening Contract/Relax Program

You should continue practicing your reverse Kegel program until you feel like you are gaining control over your muscles. The only way to tell if you have complete relaxation is to test your PFM by inserting a finger into your vagina and grading the release. I have created a 4-level grading system and included it in Table 4.1 so you can accurately evaluate your progress. This is the most accurate way to test because I find many of my patients think they are releasing when in reality they are contracting the muscles and creating more pain. When you test yourself, grade yourself on a scale of 1-4. A grade of 3 or 4 should be achieved before starting your Kegel strengthening contract/relax program.

What will you feel with your finger during your reverse Kegel self-grade test? You should feel the tension or grip around your finger releasing, and the finger should gently slip outward. You can also use a mirror to better visualize the reverse Kegel. When using a mirror, you should see the muscles come towards the mirror. You should also see the perineal body, or area between the vagina and the rectum, drop down towards the mirror. If you see this area lifting up, you are doing the reverse Kegel series incorrectly. Also look at your anus with the mirror. The anus should open up as if you were passing gas, but not pushing out, which is a sign of bearing down and straining. Again, if you see the anus contract and pull in, you are performing the reverse Kegel incorrectly.

Table 4.2: Reverse Kegel Downtraining Series

TECHNIQUE
1. Rose Petal Flower Release
2. Direct Vaginal Release
3. Child's Pose Release
4. Prayer Squat Release
5. Dead Bug Release
6. Mini-Squat Release
7. Side Lying Sit Bones Apart Release
8. Dropping the Panties
9. Body Check Release

Reverse Kegel Downtraining Series

Rose Petal Flower Release

WHAT TO DO:

As you breathe in for 5 to 7 seconds, send your inhalation breath to your vaginal muscles visualizing and imagining them as a large tight rose flower that is beginning to blossom in the springtime. Imagine the rose opening up petal by petal. Try this exercise for 5 breaths.

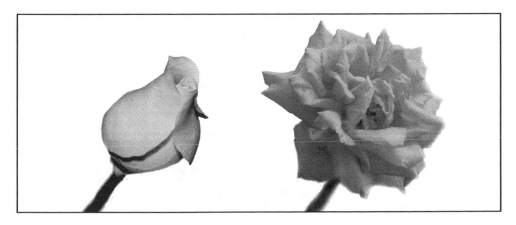

Direct Vaginal Release

WHAT TO DO:

1. Place your clean, gloved finger or dilator into your vagina. Try to find a position that is comfortable for you to maintain your finger in your vagina for at least 5 minutes. You can try different positions such as standing, sitting or lying on your side and find the one that works best for you. At times you may be able to do a PFM release in one position but not another. It is important to try all positions to enhance PFM relaxation in any position.

2. As you breathe in, send your in-breath into your vagina and imagine that the walls of your vagina are expanding away from the dilator or finger. If you are using a dilator, you should feel the dilator gently and slowly slip out of the vagina as you do your relaxation exercises.

3. If your dilator/finger is being pushed out as you do your direct release then you are forcing the release and putting undue stress and strain on your pelvic muscles. Pushing to get the release is not the same as gently allowing it to happen with your in-breath. Always couple the visualization with the inhalation.

Child's Pose Release

WHAT TO DO:

1. Go on your hands and knees and then bring your body into child's pose as in the above photo. Bring one hand onto each sit bone and keep contact with the bones as you perform your PFM relaxation child's pose release.

2. If your sit bones do not touch your heels, place a pillow under your gluteal muscles and feet. Now imagine as you breathe in for a count of 5 seconds that your sit bones are moving away from each other. Simultane-ously feel your pelvic muscles release and relax. Make sure your in-breath lasts as long as the pelvic release (at least 5 seconds), and then perform for 5 breaths.

Prayer Squat Release

WHAT TO DO:

1. Get into the Prayer Squat Position as photographed in the above photo. It's best to hold on to a sturdy object when performing this exercise to facilitate the pelvic floor muscle release and to reduce any undue stress this exercise can put on the thighs, back and calf muscles.

2. If your heels do not touch the floor, place a pillow under your heels to make this exercise more comfortable and less stressful.

3. Send your in-breath into your vaginal pelvic floor muscles for a count of 5 seconds.

4. You can remain in this position for 10 releases or you can get up and down within each repetition.

5. Aim to be in this position for 5 minutes a day.

6. While performing the exercises, focus on inhalation breathing, making sure not to hold your breath.

Dead Bug Release

WHAT TO DO:

1. Lie on your back, bring your knees to your chest and place one hand on the inside of each knee.

2. While inhaling, imagine your sit bones coming apart and your pelvic muscles releasing. Inhale for at least 5 seconds, exhale and repeat for 5 breaths.

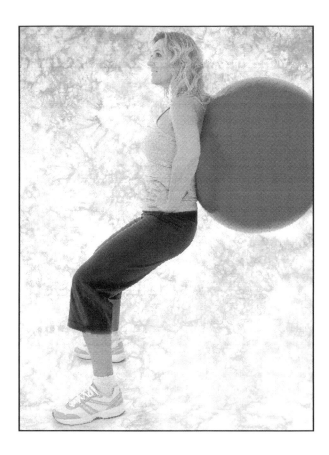

Mini-Squat Release

WHAT TO DO:

1. While standing with feet hip-width apart, knees slightly bent and in good postural alignment, place one hand on each hip bone.

2. Imagine you are about to sit in a chair and perform a mini-squat, while focusing on inhaling into your PFM and simultaneously visualizing your sit bones coming apart. Lower your body for 5 seconds as you breathe in and go back to start position as you exhale.

3. Repeat 10 times or do as many as you can tolerate. This exercise is great because it works with gravity to get you the PFM release and at the same time strengthens your legs.

Side Lying Sit Bones Apart Release

WHAT TO DO:

1. Lay down on your right side and place your left hand on your left sit bone.

2. As you breathe in, pull the left sit bone away from the right. Feel and imagine your pelvic floor muscles dropping outward, relaxing and releasing.

3. Hold this release for 5 seconds, go back to neutral or start position and repeat for 5 breaths.

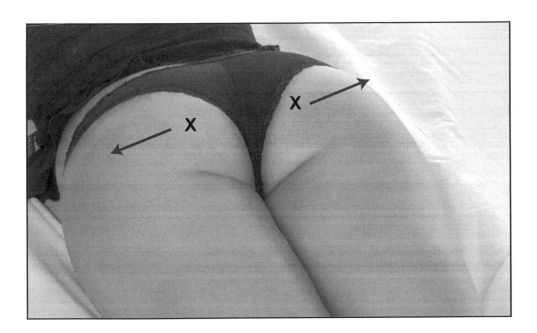

The X's represent the location of the sit bones' release. The arrows represent the way you should imagine your sit bones moving while you are in side lying position.

Dropping the Panties

WHAT TO DO:

1. Sit with good posture with your weight evenly distributed on your sit bones.

2. Practice diaphragmatic breathing for several minutes to center yourself.

3. Breathe in for a count of 5 and imagine that your panties and vaginal muscles are dropping into the chair.

4. Make sure to direct your in-breath to your PFM. With your visualization, collect your pelvic pain and imagine the pain leaving your body with your exhalation or out-breath.

Body Check Release

WHAT TO DO:

1. In any position, start with 1 to 2 minutes of diaphragmatic breathing to center yourself.

2. Tune into your muscles, and ask yourself, "Where are my muscles in space and in what state are they in?"

3. Practice releasing the muscles with the inhalation breath.

4. This technique should be utilized during stressful times such as when you are arguing with someone, and also during periods with painful flare-ups.

Traditional Kegel Contract/Relax Series

Congratulations! If you are reading this section and getting ready to move into the contract/relax series, then you are doing really well with the downtraining! Take a conscious moment to congratulate yourself for getting this far. For women in this phase of their recovery, I like to start them with a contract/relax program.

Start by examining your PFMs. Perform an internal vaginal examination with your index finger, similar to the self-grading exam for the reverse Kegels. During this self-exam you need to find out how many seconds you can hold a contraction and conversely how many seconds it takes you to release your muscles completely. These 2 numbers will determine a ratio that you will use as a starting point of your contract/relax program.

How to Determine Your Contract/Relax Program Ratio

1. Please have a mirror and lubrication on hand for your exam.

2. Start off by first looking externally at your perineum and performing a contract Kegel.

3. For correct Kegel execution look for the following motions: your clitoris should move slightly downward, your anus should wink, and the perineal body should move up and in.

4. After looking at your Kegel contraction, look at your reverse Kegel. You should see the anus release and your perineal body move outwards towards the mirror.

5. Once you are performing the Kegel and the reverse Kegel correctly, place a well-lubricated index finger into your vagina and contract your PFM around your finger. Count to see how many seconds you can hold the contraction by counting 1 Mississippi, 2 Mississippi, 3 Mississippi, etc. Stop counting once you feel the contraction of the Kegel get weaker or release. This is the number of seconds to use for the contract.

6. Start releasing your muscles and see how many counts of Mississippi it takes you to release your PFM completely. From these 2 numbers, determine your contract/relax ratio. For example, you might start out with a 5-second Kegel contraction and a 10-second release so your ratio would be 1:2.

7. Always err on the side of safety by giving yourself more time to release.

Kegel Strengthening Program

Contract/Relax and Slow/Relax

1. Now that you have determined your ratio, start your strengthening program conservatively by performing 10 repetitions of contract/relax 3 times daily, incorporating your ratio as your guide.

2. Pay close attention to make sure your pelvic pain does not increase with your current strengthening program. If you start to experience more pain, stop the contract/relax exercises immediately and go back to the relaxation exercises and/or the internal work described in Part III.

3. After 1 to 2 weeks, if you are doing well with your contract/relax program, start doing your program 4 to 5 times daily.

4. After 2 weeks, retest to see if your PFM contract endurance has improved. If it is longer, then add more seconds to your contraction Kegel. For example, after 2 weeks of diligently doing your strengthening exercises, you can now hold your slow Kegels for 7 seconds. Then start doing your program with 7 seconds contract and 14 seconds release, using the same 1:2 ratio as a guide. You may find your ratio changes over time, and if so, this is acceptable.

Quick-Flick Kegels

In conjunction with your contract/relax Kegel, add the quick-flick Kegel exercises as well. These consist of 1 to 2 second contracts followed by 1 to 2 second releases, repeated 10 to 20 times. These quick Kegels should be performed after resting for 1 minute after the slow Kegels.

For strengthening programs, the goal that I usually set for my patients is a 10-second slow Kegel contraction with a 10 to 20 second release, performed 3 to 5 times daily. After one set of the slow Kegels, I recommend waiting 1 minute and then doing 10 to 20 quick Kegels. By performing both types of Kegel strengthening exercises, you will hit the slow twitch and fast twitch muscle fibers of the pelvic floor.

Correct Kegel downtraining followed by Kegel strengthening is part of the foundation of your healing journey. As you master your Kegel program in conjunction with the self-massage and intra-vaginal techniques found in Part III of this book, you will be armed with some very powerful tools that can help you regain a pain-free life. Do not quit if you find yourself feeling frustrated with your breathing and releasing on the inhale. Be content to make small improvements if needed, in the beginning. You will achieve breakthroughs as long as you continue to persevere.

Strive for a deep understanding of your body so that you can remain aware of your PFMs with your day to day activities.

In the next chapters, you will be doing contract/relax Kegels while performing physio ball strengthening, and you will also do reverse Kegels while releasing stress at work and with your yoga program.

In Their Own Words – One Woman's Search for Answers

"My pain started 8 years ago when I had sex with a new partner. It was a pain I was unfamiliar with – burning and abrasive. My first thought was that I had a yeast infection so I consulted a nurse-midwife. She confirmed the presence of yeast and prescribed boric acid capsules especially formulated by a compounding pharmacy. I tried this as well as garlic cloves inserted as pessaries, off and on for a year or so. The pain would come and go; at times increasing dramatically with normal activities like sitting and walking to the subway. These times, I felt the pain more intensely as if being stabbed or burned.

"Realizing this was not a yeast infection, I went back to the nurse-midwife. She told me later that she suspected I had vulvodynia, but didn't want to diagnose me herself. She sent me to a respected OB/GYN in a large practice. The doctor confirmed her suspicion; but when I asked about treatment options, I was horrified. They included using novocaine to numb the area; applying estrogen cream; taking antiseizure and antidepressant drugs like Neurontin; and finally, surgery to remove the painful areas. In the meantime, the doctor recommended I have a glass of wine and try to relax the next time I had sex.

"I did not find comfort until some time later when a new OB/GYN recommended physical therapy; specifically, internal trigger point and myofascial release. She referred me to Isa's practice where I have been going for a few months now. Since starting the therapy, I see a huge improvement. Isa told me that having a dysfunctional pelvic floor for years has caused other body parts to be affected. By this time, I was also experiencing pain in my hip joints and lower back.

"So far, the result has been wonderful! Not only am I experiencing less pain, I am also learning a lot about the interconnections of the pelvis, hips and back muscles, and how to keep them all talking to each other happily through manual release of trigger points, the use of a foam roller, and stretching. I don't mind that the program has required a lot of work from me because the results are immense. It is such a relief to know there is a valid treatment for this pain. It is not just psychological, and now I have a whole arsenal of tools to stay in control of my pain."

Chapter Five

"To me, good health is more than just exercise and diet. It's really a point of view and a mental attitude you have about yourself."
— Angela Lansbury

Chapter 5

THE HERRERA PILATES BALL STRENGTHENING
ROUTINE FOR PELVIC PAIN™

Overcoming your pain and getting on the right track to long-term management of your condition requires a multidisciplined approach. One of the important disciplines you will have to undertake is to get yourself on a basic strengthening program to better align and hold your body. I have developed a great workout for my patients which I will share with you in this chapter. Based on Pilates and using the physio ball, this concentrated and focused routine targets areas that are often weakened and shut down by pelvic pain.

In the beginning, do all of the exercises in the routine. As you gain confidence and strength, mix and match to come up with your own sets and routines that give you the most targeted relief. Remember to listen to your body while doing the Pilates ball exercises. Don't overdo it too soon, especially if you are not someone who has worked out much before reading this book.

Many of the lower extremity muscles in women with pelvic pain become shortened, tight and weak. Upper body muscles also become weak, contributing to poor postural alignment and pain. To regain balance in your body you must focus on a toning and strengthening program as one of the foundational blocks from which you can achieve and maintain long-term results. An overall program that incorporates upper and lower body strengthening will balance out the weaknesses, promote a healthier body, and propel you forward with the other disciplines and techniques highlighted throughout this book.

From my experience, women who suffer from pelvic pain usually have comparable body-types and similar muscular weaknesses. It is the nature of this condition for the body to often draw inwards, creating postural issues like forward head, rounded shoulders, slouching into the lower back, and general weakness in the hips. Everything in the body is connected either directly or indirectly, so it is very important to include an overall strengthening program as one of the building blocks to your long-term recovery.

How to Purchase a Physio Ball

You will need to purchase a physio ball for the strengthening and yoga series. The balls usually come in four different sizes depending on the height of the user. Use Table 5.1 as a reference when you purchase your physio ball. In addition to doing the yoga series with the ball, I love to do basic stretches and strengthening, as well as pelvic floor muscle exercises, as it helps break the boredom. It is a great tool that will help support you if you find that a stretch or exercise is too difficult, and you will find that using the ball challenges your stabilizing muscles in unique ways.

Table 5.1: Physio Ball Height Guidelines

Height of User in Feet & Inches	Size of Ball in Centimeters
4' 7" – 5' 0"	45 cm ball
5' 1" – 5' 6"	55 cm ball
5' 7" – 6' 1"	65 cm ball
6' 2" – 6' 8"	75 cm ball

Specific Considerations for Your Pelvic Floor Muscles When Performing the Pilates Series

1. Very important! If you are still downtraining your PFMs and have not reached the contract/relax phase of your Kegel program, you can still perform the Pilates ball series to create balance and strength. If this is the case, keep your abdominals pulled in at 30% effort and fo-

cus on keeping your PFMs relaxed throughout the entire exercise series. If you are performing your contract/relax Kegels, then choose only 3 of the 10 exercises in which to perform your contract/release Kegels.

2. Make sure you do not do contract/relax on every exercise, as you will do over 100 kegels, which is too much for one session! For the other 7 exercises, keep your abdominals contracted at 30% effort and your PFMs relaxed and released.

Overall Considerations for Your Pelvic Pain Pilates Workout

1. Pay attention to your body alignment.

Many exercises require that you keep your back straight and that you sit in good ball posture. Good ball posture is actually the first exercise in the series so you get your body in the right frame of mind before you begin.

2. Pay attention to how you get off the ball.

To get off the ball, roll down until your buttocks are on the floor in order to protect your abdominals. This is especially important if you have diastasis recti of the abdominals. See the next section for information on how to test if you have diastasis recti.

3. Pay attention to your breath.

During the most difficult parts of the exercises, you will be asked to exhale. During the release part of the exercises, you will be asked to inhale.

4. Pay attention to your pelvic floor muscles.

Focus on your PFMs to make sure they are not overly tense and contracted. Whenever possible, incorporate a PFM contraction during exertion and a PFM reverse Kegel release when you return to the start position of the exercise.

5. Start with a warm-up.

Make sure that you begin your workout with a 5 to 10 minute cardio warm-up. You could briskly walk, treadmill, cycle, or any other activity that gets your blood pumping before you begin the routine.

6. Pay attention to your abdomen.

Your abdominals should be moderately engaged throughout the routine. Focus on bringing your belly button to your spine, about 30% of the way. Note that the physio ball exercises work mostly with the transverse abdominal muscles.

Specific Considerations for Abdominal Diastasis Recti Separation and The Herrera Pilates Ball Strengthening Routine for Pelvic Pain™

Diastasis Recti Abdominal (DRA) is a separation of the rectus abdominal muscle at the linea alba. The outmost abdominal muscles, called the rectus abdominus, form two halves, called right and left recti muscles. These two halves are covered by fibrous connective tissue from other muscles and join at the central seam called the linea alba. Like a zipper, these abdominal muscles can separate during pregnancy due to incorrect biomechanics or with sudden weight gains and obesity. DRA can also result by performing abdominal exercises incorrectly or by suddenly sitting up straight in bed from a horizontal laying down position, called "jackknifing."

DRA has profound effects on the function of the pelvic floor muscles. It is a well-known fact that the PFMs and the abdominals have a synergistic relationship. When DRA is present, it decreases the ability of the PFMs to contract effectively, contributing to urinary, stress and fecal incontinence. DRA leaves the abdominals in a weakened state. With less support for the pelvic organs, there is an increased chance of pelvic organ prolapse of the bladder, uterus and or rectum. When this separation is present in women with pelvic pain, the PFMs cannot function optimally which makes the contract/relax exercises more difficult than they need to be. Make sure to test for DRA as defined in the next section. I would recommend not beginning the Pilates series until your DRA is two fingers or less.

It is also important to note that the function and insertion of the other abdominal muscles, called the transverse and internal/external oblique is hindered when you have a DRA. This altered state in the abdominals can lead to the formation of trigger points in the abdominal wall. These abdominal trigger points can cause urinary urgency, urinary frequency, pelvic pain and pelvic pressure. Many times these abdominal trigger points can lead to pain above the pubic bone and can cause the sensations of urinary tract infections (UTI), without actually having UTI . Not only does the DRA need to be corrected but also all abdominal trigger points need to be resolved. Use the techniques outlined in Part III of this book to eliminate trigger points.

First, you must determine if you have a DRA by performing the test on page 79 and then you must do the corrective exercises to close the gap. See pages 80 to 82 for exercises to correct your DRA, one seated and one lying down on your back. If you have very weak abdominal muscles, start with the seated exercise and then incorporate the lying down corrective exercise in one week. It takes time to close up a DRA separation. It requires that you are consistent with the exercises and that you consider the "Tips to Avoid Making the DRA Worse" on page 80.

Diastasis Recti

Recti Abdominus Muscles

Tracking DRA

Use this chart to keep track of your progress as you work to close your DRA.

Table 5.2: DRA Tracking

DATE	2 INCHES ABOVE	AT UMBILICUS	2 INCHES BELOW

How to Test for DRA Separation

1. Lie on your back with your knees bent.

2. Exhale and slightly lift your upper back off the floor with your arms reaching forward. Check how many fingers you are able to insert horizontally two inches above the umbilicus, at the umbilicus, and two inches below the umbilicus.

3. DRA of one to two fingers separation is considered normal. A three-finger separation requires correction. Corrective exercises are used to close up any separation of the abdominals.

Tips to Avoid Making the DRA Worse

1. Avoid jackknifing out of bed. Instead, logroll out of bed by engaging your abdominals, turning completely to the side and then use your arms to push yourself to a seated position.

2. Avoid sudden weight gains especially during pregnancy.

3. Avoid yoga exercises that stretch the abdominals such as the "Ball Wheel" highlighted in Chapter 6 on page 119.

4. Avoid coughing or sneezing without first engaging your abdominals.

5. Avoid traditional abdominal exercises such as the abdominal crunches which can make the DRA larger.

6. Avoid exercises at the gym or daily activities that make your belly pop out. New moms should be careful with pushing strollers and lifting their children.

Corrective DRA Exercises: Seated Splinted Head Raises

WHAT TO DO:

1. Sit in cross-legged position with correct posture, shoulders over hips.

2. Crisscross your hands over your belly, or use a scarf or Dyna-Band to bring the abdominals together.

3. Inhale through your nose into your belly. Exhale through your mouth to

initiate the belly button reaching towards the spine, engaging the abdominals.

4. Simultaneously, pull the sides of your abdominal together with your arms to approximate the recti muscles. You can also do a gentle PFM contraction while doing this exercise.

5. Breathe naturally and hold for 5 seconds. Return to start position.

6. Perform 20 times, 2 to 3 times a day.

Corrective DRA Exercises: Lying Down Splinted Head Raises

WHAT TO DO:

1. Lie on your back with your knees bent on the floor.

2. Bring your belly button to your spine and press your lower back into the floor.

3. Crisscross your hands over your belly, or use a scarf or Dyna-Band to bring the abdominals together.

4. Exhale very slowly, contract your abdominals and raise your head toward your chest just before the diastasis bulge begins. Keep the shoulders in contact with the floor to begin. To maximize the approximation of the recti mucles you can use a large scarf or wrap to bring the muscles together. You can also do a gentle PFM contraction while doing this exercise.

5. Breathe naturally and hold for 5 seconds. Return to start position. As you get stronger, you will be able to lift your shoulders off the floor.

6. Perform 20 times, 2 to 3 times a day.

Once you have become aware of your diastasis and have begun to take corrective measures, you will be ready to move ahead into the Pilates series.

Overall Benefits of the Pilates Ball Series

1. Your body will become strong without creating the muscle bulk that lifting traditional weights will do.

2. You will feel more flexible and buoyant, have more energy, and improve joint mobility and range of motion.

3. You will find it easier to remain in a state of good posture.

4. You will have strong abdominals without creating trigger points that are commonly found in females with pelvic pain.

5. You will be better able to discern the overall state of your pelvic floor muscles. The Pilates ball series teaches you how to exercise correctly using both the core muscles and the PFM simultaneously.

Table 5.3: The Herrera Pilates Ball Strengthening Routine for Pelvic Pain™
PDF version of this table available at http://www.Renew-PT.com

EXERCISE
1. Seated Ball Posture
2. Seated Ball Marching
3. Arm Circles on Your Back
4. Seated Ball Scapular Squeezes
5. Ball Squats
6. Ball Inner Thigh Squeezes
7. Ball Bridging
8. Alternating Arm and Leg Lifts
9. Ball Plank Side Flutter Kicks
10. Ball Push-Ups

The Herrera Pilates Ball Strengthening Routine for Pelvic Pain™

Seated Ball Posture

WHAT TO DO:

1. Sit tall on the ball with your weight evenly distributed on your sit bones, ears aligned with the shoulders, and abdominal muscles pulled in.

2. Your knees and hips should form a right angle with your feet flat on the floor. It's acceptable for your hips to be slightly higher than your knees, but not the other way around because it will put stress on your lower back and leg muscles.

3. Pull your shoulder blades back towards each other; imagine you are putting your shoulder blades into your back pockets, in and down.

5. Once comfortably in this posture, practice 5 to 10 minutes of diaphragmatic breathing together with reverse Kegels or contract/relax Kegels, depending on where you are in your Kegel program as defined in Chapter 4.

6. This is called "good ball posture" and is the basis of many of the exercises in this series.

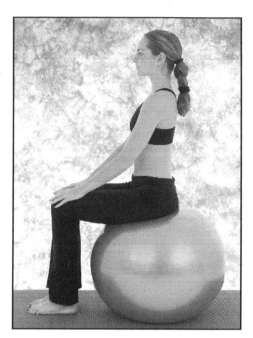

WHAT TO WATCH OUT FOR:

1. Incorrect ball size will put increased pressure and strain on muscles. Use Table 5.1 on page 75 to determine which ball is the proper size for your height.

2. Avoid rounding the shoulders or lower back and sticking your chin out, as these will cause pain or strain to your body and could lead to injury.

BENEFITS:

1. Provides good sensory input for the reverse and contract/relax Kegel exercises, as your PFMs are in direct contact with the surface of the ball.

2. Reinforces good sitting posture which will help decrease pain associated with poor sitting and/or slouching at work or home.

Seated Ball Marching

WHAT TO DO:

1. Sit on the center of the ball with good ball posture, with feet hip-width apart and with hands on the ball for added support.

2. Exhale, contract abdominals and PFMs, and then raise the right leg about 2 to 3 inches from the floor. Hold for 2 seconds.

3. Inhale, relax PFMs, and lower the foot. Switch sides, alternating the foot lifts until you have completed 10 repetitions on both sides.

RECOMMENDED STRETCH AFTER THIS EXERCISE:

Ball Warrior Two as detailed in the yoga series in Chapter 6 on page 120.

WHAT TO WATCH OUT FOR:

1. Avoid slouching the lower back and rounding the shoulder blades.

2. Avoid shifting too much weight to the supported foot. Try to keep your weight evenly distributed on your sit bones, hands, and supported foot.

BENEFITS:

1. Strengthens core muscles and leg muscles.

2. Improves balance and posture.

3. Connects you to your PFMs and helps you to contract and relax the pelvic floor muscles.

Arm Circles on Your Back

WHAT TO DO:

1. Sit with good ball posture on the center of the ball.

2. Walk your feet in front of you until your thighs are parallel to the floor and your upper back and head rest comfortably on the ball.

3. Place your arms by the side of your legs, remembering not to collapse into your lower back but keeping the back straight and lifted.

4. Inhale, relax the PFMs, and raise your arms over your head as in the photo.

5. Exhale, contract your PFMs and abdominal muscles, and roll your arms out to the side, finishing with your arms by your legs, creating a circle motion. This is one cycle.

6. Do 10 cycles.

7. When you are finished with this exercise, relax on the floor. Lie down on your back and hug your knees into your chest to release the lower back muscles if they are tight.

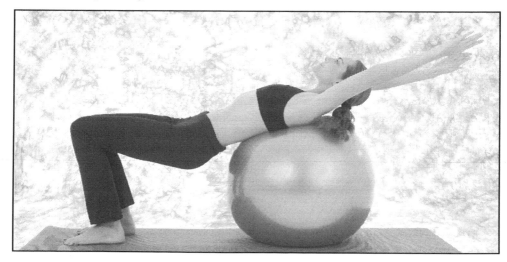

RECOMMENDED STRETCH AFTER THIS EXERCISE:

Seated 4 Stretch as detailed in the workplace series in Chapter 7 on page 134. This can be performed on the ball.

WHAT TO WATCH OUT FOR:

1. Avoid slumping in the lower back area. Your lower back should be straight and parallel to your thighs.

2. If your shoulders are too tight to perform the arm circles, skip the circles and extend your arms straight up instead of over your head and then lower them to the side.

3. Keep the shoulder blades pulled together and stabilized on the ball and do not raise them up with the arm circles.

BENEFITS:

1. Strengthens the lower back, gluteal, abdominals, and hamstring muscles.

2. Strengthens the core abdominal muscles and also the arm muscles.

3. Helps improve posture by improving arm range of motion and stretching the chest muscles.

4. Helps to strengthen and relax the pelvic floor muscles.

Seated Ball Scapular Squeezes

WHAT TO DO:

1. Sit with good ball posture with arms reaching forward and palms resting on the front of the thighs.

2. Exhale, contract the abdominals and PFMs, and rotate your palms out. Bring your arms back until your hands are in alignment with the sides of your body.

3. Simultaneously bring your shoulder blades towards each other, and imagine them sliding down your back and into your back pockets. Breathe naturally and hold 3 to 5 seconds.

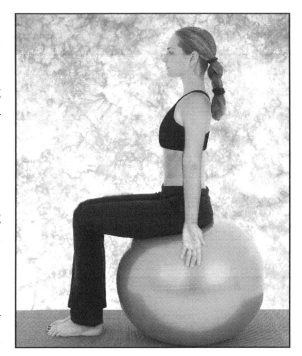

4. Inhale, release the PFM, and rotate your arms and palms back to the start position. Repeat 10 times.

RECOMMENDED STRETCH AFTER THIS EXERCISE:

Seated Side Stretch as detailed in the workplace series in Chapter 7 on page 132. This can also be performed on the physio ball.

WHAT TO WATCH OUT FOR:

1. Avoid slouching the upper and lower back muscles.

2. Do not stick your chin out. Make sure your chin is tucked back at all times.

3. Be sure to keep your chest forward and your shoulder blades back and down.

BENEFITS:

1. Improves posture by strengthening the rhomboideous and lower trap muscles.

2. Encourages PFMs to become toned, strengthened and relaxed.

3. Stretches chest muscles and improves upper body flexibility.

Ball Squats

WHAT TO DO:

1. Place your physio ball against a wall and lean against it with the small of your back touching the ball. Maintain your abdominals slightly engaged with this exercise. Focus on bringing your belly button to your spine, about 30 percent of the effort. Walk your feet forward slightly, allowing your knees to be in a 90-degree angle when you execute the squat.

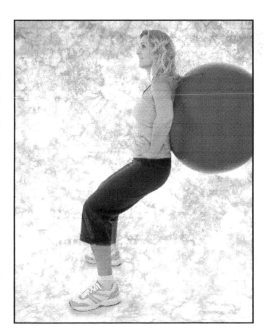

2. Inhale, relax the PFMs, and lower your body until your thighs are parallel to the floor, forming a 90-degree angle. Make sure your knees are on top of your ankles and your back is straight. Hold for 2 to 5 seconds.

3. Exhale, contract your PFMs, and raise yourself to your original position. Repeat 10 times.

RECOMMENDED STRETCH AFTER THIS EXERCISE:

Hamstring on Wall Pose as detailed in the yoga series in Chapter 6 on page 112.

WHAT TO WATCH OUT FOR:

1. Avoid lowering the buttocks lower than the knees, as this will strain your knee ligaments and lower back muscles.

2. Do not let your knees pass your ankles to avoid straining your knees.

3. Watch out for poor breath and PFM coordination.

BENEFITS:

1. Strengthens main muscle groups that become weak in women with pelvic pain, including quadriceps, hamstring, gluteal, inner and outer thigh muscles.

2. Helps maintain correct bio-mechanics because the legs are strong enough to participate in lifting motions.

3. Strengthens and relaxes the PFMs.

Ball Inner Thigh Squeezes

WHAT TO DO:

1. Lie on your left side, with left knee bent and right leg straight up on the ball, as in photo.

2. Exhale, squeeze your abdominals and PFMs, while simultaneously pressing your right leg into the ball for 5 seconds.

3. Inhale, release the downward pressure on the ball from your leg. Then release the PFMs for 5 seconds, and perform a reverse Kegel as outlined in Chapter 4.

4. Repeat 10 times, then switch sides.

RECOMMENDED STRETCH AFTER THIS EXERCISE:

Wall V Stretch as detailed in the yoga series in Chapter 6 on page 111.

WHAT TO WATCH OUT FOR:

1. Be careful to accurately perform the proper contract/relax for your pelvic floor muscles while doing this exercise as you can easily create muscle spasms if the exercise is done incorrectly.

2. Make sure to stretch after this exercise to prevent trigger points in the inner thigh muscles.

BENEFITS:

1. Tones and strengthens the inner thigh muscles creating balance in the pelvic-hip muscles.

2. Strengthens the PFMs.

3. Can improve leg, foot, ankle and knee alignment for better walking posture.

Ball Bridging

WHAT TO DO:

1. Lie on your back and place your heels on top of the physio ball. Allow your head, shoulders, and arms to relax into the floor.

2. Keeping your legs slightly bent and feet pointing up, exhale and lift your hips up off the floor while simultaneously doing a PFM contraction. Hold this position for 2 to 5 seconds.

3. Inhale and lower your hips slowly while simultaneously performing a reverse Kegel. Hold this position for 5 seconds.

4. Repeat the up and down movement 10 times.

5. If needed, stretch your lower back by gently hugging your knees to your chest.

RECOMMENDED STRETCH AFTER THIS EXERCISE:

Pretzel Pose as detailed in the yoga series in Chapter 6 on page 116.

WHAT TO WATCH OUT FOR:

1. Avoid holding the breath and tensing the shoulders and neck muscles.

2. If you are unable to perform a contract/relax Kegel, focus on the lifting and lowering phase of the bridge.

3. Stop immediately if this exercise produces pain in the lower back or neck muscles.

4. If you experience hamstring soreness, stretch your hamstrings using the Hamstring on Wall Pose found in Chapter 6 on page 112.

BENEFITS:

1. Strengthens core and pelvic floor muscles in addition to the gluteal, hamstrings, and inner thighs.

2. Helps improve lower back spinal alignment.

Alternating Arm and Leg Lifts

WHAT TO DO:

1. Lie on your stomach, facedown on your physio ball, maintaining a good

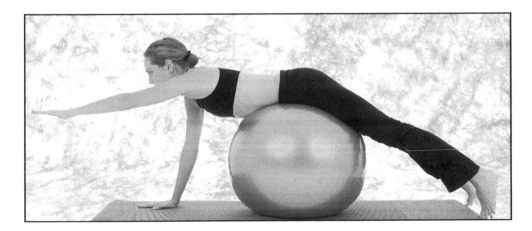

balance between upper and lower body with hands and toes on the floor for added support.

2. Keep hands and feet shoulder-width apart, with your shoulder blades pulled towards each other and your abdominals contracted.

3. Exhale, contract PFMs, and raise your left arm straight out until it is level with your ear.

4. Inhale, relax the PFMs, lower your left arm to the floor, and switch arms. Repeat 10 times on each side.

5. For an additional challenge, raise your right arm and left leg simultaneously. Hold for 2 seconds and then lower both limbs. Repeat with the left arm and right leg.

RECOMMENDED STRETCH AFTER THIS EXERCISE:

Pigeon pose as detailed in the yoga series in Chapter 6 on page 110.

WHAT TO WATCH OUT FOR:

1. The ball will wobble in the beginning as you get used to this exercise. Perform the exercise slowly to help maintain ball stability.

2. Avoid overarching the back and raising the arms and legs too high.

3. Do not raise your hips off the ball as you raise the legs up.

BENEFITS:

1. Strengthens lower back, arms, shoulders, and hip muscles.

2. Improves posture and core strength.

3. Improves PFM strength, relaxation, and coordination.

Ball Plank Side Flutter Kicks

WHAT TO DO:

1. Lie on your stomach, facedown on your physio ball with palms resting on the floor.

2. Walk your hands and body forward until the ball is at your upper thighs. Make sure to keep your hands a little wider than shoulder-width apart and your feet together.

3. Exhale, contract the PFMs and abdominals, and bring your legs out to the side a little wider than hip-width apart for 3 to 5 seconds. Be careful not to hyper-extend or round your back.

4. Inhale, release the PFMs, and bring your legs back to starting position. Relax for 3 to 5 seconds, then repeat 10 times.

5. For an extra challenge, add a Dyna-Band around your ankles to make the outward movement of your legs more difficult. A Dyna-Band is an elastic band with different color-coded resistance. Start with the easiest resistance and progress as tolerated.

RECOMMENDED STRETCH AFTER THIS EXERCISE:

Knee Down Twist pose as detailed in the yoga series in Chapter 6 on page 108.

WHAT TO WATCH OUT FOR:

1. Avoid hyper-extending your elbows, which will put strain and stress on the ligaments.

2. Keep your neck in alignment with the rest of your spine and avoid sticking your jaw out.

3. Avoid sagging in the lower back which could potentially hurt your spine.

4. Be careful of wrist and hand pain.

BENEFITS:

1. Strengthens the outer thighs, gluteal muscles, arms and shoulders.

2. Improves core and PFM strength, relaxation and coordination.

Ball Push-Ups

WHAT TO DO:

1. Lie on your stomach, facedown on your physio ball with palms resting on the floor.

2. Walk your hands and body forward until the ball is at your shins, as in the photo below. Make sure to keep your feet together and your hands a little wider than shoulder-width apart. To make it a bit easier, only walk your body forward to your upper thighs.

3. Inhale, relax the PFMs, bend your arms and lower your body until your elbows are aligned with your shoulders, making a right angle.

4. Exhale, contract the PFMs and abdominals, and straighten out the arms and elbows without hyper-extending the elbows. Repeat 10 times.

RECOMMENDED STRETCH AFTER THIS EXERCISE:

Seated Chest Opener as detailed in the workplace series in Chapter 7 on page 139. This can be performed on the physio ball.

WHAT TO WATCH OUT FOR:

1. If it is too difficult to lower your body all the way, do baby push-ups by not lowering the body too much.

2. Avoid hyper-extending your elbows, which will put strain and stress on the ligaments.

3. Keep your neck in alignment with the rest of your spine and avoid sticking your jaw out.

4. Avoid sagging in the lower back which could potentially hurt your spine.

5. Be careful of wrist and hand pain. Keep your body weight evenly distributed among all 5 fingers and imagine that you are pushing the floor away from you as you raise your body up.

BENEFITS:

1. Strengthens the chest and increases the endurance of the shoulders and arm muscles.

2. Improves core and PFM strength.

Now that you have become familiar with the key aspects of the strengthening series, let's take a look at the yoga series in the next chapter, which is the perfect compliment to your conditioning program.

Chapter Six

"Happiness cannot be traveled to, owned, earned
worn, or consumed. Happiness is the spiritual experience
of living every minute with love, grace, and gratitude."
— *Dennis Waitley*

Chapter 6

THE HERRERA YOGA SERIES FOR PELVIC PAIN™

The essential stretches highlighted in this chapter help stretch the outer pelvic hip muscles, the lower back, the gluteal muscles and abdominal muscles, all of which are intimately connected with your PFMs. By stretching these adjacent, outer pelvic and hip muscles, you are indirectly releasing tension in the PFMs. The poses in this yoga series were chosen because I found that when these were incorporated into their treatment programs, my patients felt less overall pain and the yoga series helped control the intensity of their flare-ups. My patients tell me that when they have painful flare-ups, this yoga series is a lifesaver. Many of my patients have also told me that the stretching helped to release the tension and tightness they feel in their pelvic, lower back and hip muscles.

The series also indirectly helps you feel more relaxed and calm. Many patients also report that after consistently performing the yoga series they are able to insert their dilators more easily and perform their intra-vaginal stretching, trigger point and myofascial releases with less difficulty and with less pain. Do not worry if you have not done yoga before. The series can be performed by most women even if stretching is entirely new. Remember to be content to "be" just where you are that day, not allowing yourself to get discouraged if you discover an extremely difficult and painful stretch.

When my patients perform the stretching poses highlighted in this chapter while hooked up to computerized biofeedback sensors, their pelvic floor muscle resting baseline outputs are reduced. The resting baseline seen with biofeedback represents the activity in the pelvic floor muscles at rest. At rest, the baseline should appear flat, smooth and should register under two microvolts. But in women with sexual and pelvic pain, resting biofeedback levels are often erratic and tremendously higher than two microvolts. I frequently use biofeedback as a tool to treat sexual pain and pelvic pain because it allows my patients to visualize muscles that are difficult to see, allowing them to tune in to these areas.

The exercises in this chapter are yoga-based. I recommend that they be performed in sequential order; these poses were written in this order so that you can flow into and out of the poses with ease. However, once you have mastered the series, you can perform just the poses that give you the most pain relief. Think of it as your own vaginal pelvic yoga class.

While performing the exercises, always stay in tune with your pelvic floor muscles. Ask yourself, "Do my pelvic floor muscles feel uptight or relaxed and loose?" With all the stretches, you should keep your focus on maintaining relaxed and released PFMs. Many of the stretches in this chapter are intense and may cause you pain while you are performing them. Try to perform the stretches only to the point where you feel a mild stretch. Stretching too vigorously can lead to an increase in muscle soreness and can increase the tension in the pelvic floor muscles, resulting in heightened pelvic pain. Keep your mind focused on the stretches and do not let your mind wander to what you have to do today at work or what chores you need to do. It is important to stay connected with all the sensations you are feeling and especially important to avoid holding your breath. Holding your breath, also called valsalva, will strain and excessively stress your pelvic floor muscles.

Let this stretching series become an integral part of your transformational body work, and you will feel better both physically and mentally afterwards.

The Herrera Yoga Series Program Guidelines

1. All stretches should be held for 10 to 60 seconds depending on your tolerance and pain.

2. The basic yoga core series should be done in its entirety as you become accustomed to the moves. As you get more used to the series, you can choose parts that are more effective for your particular needs and customize your program.

3. For better results and for pain reduction it is best to perform the yoga series up to three times per week (e.g., Monday, Wednesday, and Friday).

4. While performing the series, practice Tension Release Breathing or TRB. To understand TRB in your mind's eye, send your in-breath or inhalation to the part of your muscles where you feel the most tension or pain. Imagine that you are collecting the tension in your muscles with your in-breath. With your out-breath, exhale all the tension out of the muscles. You will learn to relax and ease the tension in your muscles much easier by performing the stretches with proper breathing techniques. I find that the patients who use this type of breathing with their stretching are able to control their pain better, especially during muscle flare-ups.

5. Make the length of your inhalation breath equal to the length of your exhalation. For instance breathe in for a count of 4 and exhale for a count of 4.

6. Try to release your PFM while you inhale. This may seem counterintuitive at first, but by doing this you will actually be working with the natural rhythm of the organs when breathing. Upon inhalation, the diaphragm drops down naturally, so try to let the PFM release as well. My patients typically have some difficulty mastering this release technique, so don't worry if this happens to you. The important thing is to focus on the PFM. If you can get a release with the exhale only at first, this is fine as well.

7. Never go beyond the stretching limit of your muscles. You should feel a mild stretch while in the poses. Stretching too deeply can lead to muscle strain, micro-tears, muscle pulls, and joint problems. All stretches are static and require that you hold them at the end position without moving. Never bounce in the stretch as you could pull or strain a muscle. This is called ballistic stretching, and it is not recommended for women suffering from pelvic pain.

8. Always get out of your stretches mindfully and slowly.

9. Start with the complete core series at first to help you gain confidence. You can then customize your poses to enhance your healing. If there are muscles that feel tighter and more tense, focus your energy on stretches that target that particular muscle.

10. For women who are inflexible or who have never stretched on a regular basis, I recommend that you hold the poses for less time until you build up your momentum.

11. The key is to pay attention to your body and observe the sensations created in your body during your yoga practice. Stay in the moment with all stretching exercises.

12. The last 4 poses of the yoga series require a a physio ball. See Chapter 5, page 75 for details on how to purchase a physio ball for your body type.

Table 6.1: The Herrera Yoga Series for Pelvic Pain™ Pose Flow Chart
PDF version of this table available at http://www.Renew-PT.com

NAME OF POSE OR STRETCH
1. Corpse Pose (start)
2. Goddess Pose
3. Knee Down Twist
4. Pigeon
5. Wall V Stretch
6. Hamstring on Wall Pose
7. Mermaid Stretch
8. Ankle to Knee
9. Pretzel Pose
10. Z Stretch
11. Ball Wheel
12. Warrior Two on Ball
13. Ball Child's Pose
14. Prayer Squat
15. Corpse Pose (end)

Corpse Pose

WHAT TO DO:

1. Lie on your back with your legs straight and arms relaxed out to the side, palms facing up. Feel your belly rise gently when you inhale and feel your belly lower when you exhale.

2. Now bring your awareness to your PFMs and direct your inhalation into this area. With your mind's eye, see and feel your PFMs let go and release as you breathe in. When you exhale, release the stress, tension and pain held in the body.

3. If your mind wanders, say the word release and bring your awareness back to your breathing.

4. Practice your reverse Kegels in this pose as outlined in Chapter 4, page 61.

WHAT TO WATCH OUT FOR:

1. Be careful not to hold your breath and do not push the muscles out.

2. If you cannot release the PFMs when you inhale, do not worry. You can also focus on PFM release on the exhale until you have learned to release them on the inhale. Remember, your diaphragm goes down on the in-breath, so focus on dropping the PFMs in conjunction with your diaphragm.

BENEFITS:

1. Reduces pelvic/vaginal muscle tension.

2. Relieves pelvic pain.

3. Reduces stress.

4. Quiets the mind.

5. Stretches inner thigh/groin muscles which are intimately connected to the PFM.

Goddess Pose

WHAT TO DO:

1. Lie on your back and place the soles of your feet together. Allow the weight of your legs to pull your knees toward the floor.

2. You will feel a gentle stretch and release on your inner thigh muscles.

3. Breathe diaphragmatically as you feel your inner thigh muscles release. This is also a great pose in which to practice your daily meditation and reverse Kegels.

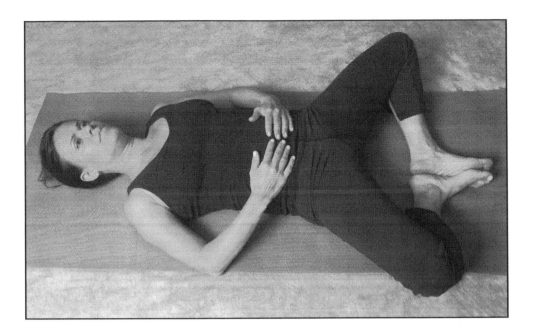

WHAT TO WATCH OUT FOR:

1. Strain on the inner thighs will be felt by women with tight muscles in this area. To make this exercise more comfortable, if you are feeling excessive strain or pain, place one to two pillows under each knee for added support.

2. If you experience discomfort in the sacroiliac joint or lower back area, place one to two pillows under your knees for added support and to reduce stress in the lower back.

BENEFITS:

1. Inner thigh muscles are frequently tight in women with pelvic pain and are often filled with trigger points that can refer pain to the pelvic floor and even elicit symptoms of urinary urgency. This intimate relationship is sometimes overlooked but these important muscles can actually contribute to overall pelvic misalignment.

2. The Goddess Pose is a great stress-releasing position to do your trigger

point releases and to massage the groin, inner thigh, and labias. This pose is also good for external PFM stretching, as highlighted in Part III of this book.

Knee Down Twist

WHAT TO DO:

1. Lie on your back and grab your right knee with your left hand, keeping your right hand extended out to the side as in the photo. Gently bring your right knee across your body until the right knee makes contact with the floor, if possible.

2. Your lower back will come off the floor, creating a spinal twisting motion. Focus your gaze on your outstretched right hand.

3. You may hear or feel a spinal release, as this pose can elicit a gentle spinal adjustment.

4. Repeat on the other side.

WHAT TO WATCH OUT FOR:

1. Avoid pulling the leg across the body too vigorously and creating nerve pain and or lower back pain.

2. Do not hold your breath as this is an intense stretch.

3. If you experience excessive pain in your lower back muscles or tailbone, you might be forcing the knee down to the floor too hard. Your lumbar spine may also have restrictions and you may find that this stretch is not appropriate for you in the beginning.

4. If you feel pain traveling down the leg, stop immediately.

BENEFITS:

1. Enhances proper nerve function and blood supply for a healthier vagina, rectum, and pelvic muscles.

2. The twisting motion compresses your organs, so when you release the pose, fresh blood and energy flows into your organs.

3. Helps decrease pelvic congestion.

Pigeon

WHAT TO DO:

1. Get on all fours with your knees below your hips and your hands underneath your shoulders.

2. Bring the left knee forward until it touches the right wrist; keep the left leg straight back behind you.

3. Try to move your right foot until it is directly below your left hip. If this is not possible, keep the foot back.

4. Keep your hips squared and level.

5. With your arms straight, support your torso. If you are very flexible, support your torso while resting on your elbows.

6. Keep your gaze straight ahead. If you are resting on your elbows, you can drop the head down.

7. Use a folded blanket or pillow under your right buttock if you have trouble lowering the hips evenly.

8. Switch sides and repeat.

WHAT TO WATCH OUT FOR:

1. Do not force yourself into this pose as it will strain your knees and hips.

2. Avoid tensing the pelvic floor muscles while in this pose.

BENEFITS:

1. Opens up the hip flexors and hip rotators which are commonly tight in women with pelvic pain.

2. Promotes hip and lower back flexibility.

Wall V Stretch

WHAT TO DO:

1. Lie face up near a wall with your buttocks as close to the wall as possible, and your legs up the wall.

2. Keep your hips and lower back flat on the floor.

3. Keep your body relaxed while you move both feet apart from each other.

4. Only open your legs until you feel a mild to medium stretch in your inner thigh muscles.

WHAT TO WATCH OUT FOR:

1. Avoid pulling the legs apart with too much force as this could lead to an inner-groin or leg muscle pull or strain. Keep this stretch gentle and avoid

pulling the thighs out too vigorously which can create pain with the stretch.

2. Many times pain during this stretch can translate to more tension in the pelvic floor muscles. It is extremely important to be aware of any increased tension in the PFMs and to release it while performing this stretch.

BENEFITS:

1. Increases flexibility in the inner thigh muscles and creates an overflow releasing effect to the pelvic floor muscles.

2. Indirectly helps to stretch out the skin and any scar present in the perineum, enhancing scar mobility.

Hamstring on Wall Pose

WHAT TO DO:

1. Lie face up near a wall with your buttocks facing the wall.

2. Place your hands under your knees and bring your knees to your chest. Pause here if needed for a nice lower back stretch.

3. Scoot your buttocks as close to the wall as possible.

4. Straighten out your left leg against the wall while maintaining the right leg bent against your chest.

5. Straigthen the right knee until a stretch is felt in the hamstring muscle.

6. Hold and then repeat on the other side.

WHAT TO WATCH OUT FOR:

1. Avoid straightening the knee with too much vigor and force as this can result in lower back pain or a micro-tear of the hamstring muscle.

2. Prevent your lower back from overarching. Keep your lumbar spine flat against the floor.

BENEFITS:

1. Stretching the hamstring muscle helps keep the pelvis in good alignment and improve posture.

2. Helps prevent lower back pain and excessive tension in the hips, pelvis and PFM.

3. Helps stretch out the area through which the pudenal, sciatic, and obturator nerve travel. These nerves are important for PFM health, pelvic sensation, and pelvic motion.

Mermaid Stretch

WHAT TO DO:

1. Sit with both legs bent to the right side and hold on to the top leg, as in the photo.

2. Lift the left arm upwards and gently bend to the right side until a stretch is felt in the left side muscles.

3. Hold and then repeat on the other side.

WHAT TO WATCH OUT FOR:

1. Imagine your outstretched arm touching the ceiling before you reach over.

2. Avoid compressing into the sides as this can cause pain in the lower back and side muscles.

BENEFITS:

1. Stretches the side muscles, including the quadratus lumborum or QL, latissimus dorsi, and intercostal muscles, while simultaneously improving spinal movement.

2. Improves nerve function and creates better rib mobility, enhancing diaphragmatic breathing.

Ankle to Knee

WHAT TO DO:

1. Sit tall on your sit bones and place your right ankle slightly off your left knee and place your left ankle under your right knee as in photo.

2. If you cannot get your legs to create two right angles, don't worry; slide your lower leg towards your buttocks.

3. Keeping your back straight, try to walk your fingertips forward.

4. To advance the pose, reach up and over with your right hand.

5. Repeat, crossing your legs the other way.

6. You may feel an intense stretch in the gluteal muscles of your top leg. Listen to your body, modify first and then consider getting out of the pose if the pain is too much.

7. To take it a step further, send your in-breath to the place in your hips that you feel the most tension and with your out-breath release the tension out of the hips.

8. For fantastic pain relief, massage the gluteal muscles of your top leg with your hands while in this pose.

WHAT TO WATCH OUT FOR:

1. Stay in a pain-free range as this is a difficult stretch that can cause some stretching pain. Staying within a pain-free range will avoid overflowing the tension to your hips.

2. Avoid holding your breath.

3. Put a small folded towel under your lower ankle if there is pain.

4. Make sure to keep both sit bones on the floor and equally distribute your weight on them.

BENEFITS:

This stretch completely opens up the hips and gluteal muscles. By increasing the flexibility of your hips, you get better blood flow to the pelvic organs and you will also enhance nerve function.

Pretzel Pose

WHAT TO DO:

1. Sit tall on your sit bones with your back straight.

2. Place the right knee over the left knee as in photo.

3. Keeping your back straight, try to walk your fingertips forward.

4. To advance the pose, reach up and over with your right hand.

5. Repeat, crossing your legs the other way.

WHAT TO WATCH OUT FOR:

1. Keep your back straight.

2. Sit high on your sit bones and keep your weight evenly distributed on both buttock cheeks.

3. Don't hold your breath.

BENEFITS:

1. Helps eliminate spasms and trigger points in the hip muscles.

2. Increases hip flexibility.

Z Stretch

WHAT TO DO:

1. Sit with the soles of your feet together, and then bring the right leg behind you, keeping your left leg in the same position. Your legs will create a "Z' shape.

2. Place your palms gently on your knees, focusing on keeping your back straight.

3. Switch sides and repeat.

WHAT TO WATCH OUT FOR:

If you experience knee or hip pain, bring the back leg forward.

BENEFITS:

1. Stretches hips, groin, and inner thigh muscles.

2. Improves postural alignment, helping your body maintain erect posture.

Ball Wheel

WHAT TO DO:

1. Lie with your back flat on the ball and walk your body back until the palms of your hands are directly behind you on the floor, as in the photo.

2. If this position is too intense, modify it so that you do not put your palms on the floor. Just roll back until you stretch in your abdominals, chest, and

throughout the front of your body.

WHAT TO WATCH OUT FOR:

This is a very intense position. If your back does not have the flexibility to get into this pose, be gentle with yourself. Over time this pose will help relieve your stress and calm your mind in addition to being a great stretch

BENEFITS:

1. Serves as a great stress reliever.

2. Opens up muscles which become tight due to chronic poor posture and slouching.

Warrior Two on Ball

WHAT TO DO:

1. Place physio ball under your buttocks for support.

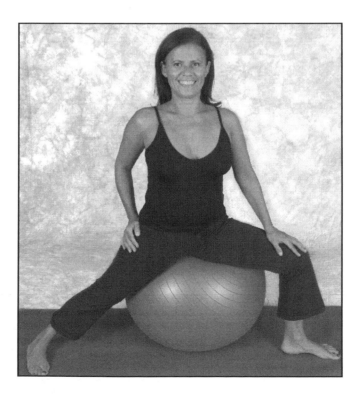

2. Bring your feet about 3 to 4 feet apart.

3. Turn your left foot out to open up the left leg, so that the left knee is over the ankle.

4. Rotate your right foot in slightly to create a 45-degree angle between your left and right foot. These angles can vary depending on the flexibility of your hips.

5. Inhale, raise your arms out to the side and look over your left shoulder. Keeping your shoulders and hips facing forward, externally rotate your hips open until you feel a stretch in your hips, inner thighs, and groin. Hold, breathe several cycles and then switch sides.

WHAT TO WATCH OUT FOR:

1. Avoid allowing your bent knee to go past 90 degrees, which would allow your knees to go past your toes as this can create knee pain and strain the knee ligaments.

2. Avoid leaning backwards and putting stress on the lower back muscles.

BENEFITS:

1. Opens up the anterior hip, through which pelvic blood supply and nerves travel, increasing blood flow and improving nerve function.

2. Increases the flexibility of the groin, hips, and inner thigh muscles.

3. Helps relieve back pain, improves balance and strengthens the legs.

Ball Child's Pose:

WHAT TO DO:

1. Get onto your hands and knees with pointed toes. Bring your buttocks towards your heels, lowering your chest towards the floor.

2. Place your hands outstretched on the ball as in the photo.

3. If this stretch is too intense, place your hands next to your body with palms up.

4. For a deeper stretch, gently roll your outstretched arms and trunk to the right, then to the left, then to neutral, using the ball to guide your motion. This is called the Angled Child's Pose.

WHAT TO WATCH OUT FOR:

1. If you feel pain in the ankles, use a pillow under your feet.

2. If your chest cannot reach the floor or you have pain or discomfort, fold a blanket or towel and place this between your buttocks and legs to give yourself additional support.

3. If you have preexisting knee conditions and experience pain in the knees with this pose, try the blanket and towel. If the pain persists, this pose might not be appropriate for you.

BENEFITS:

1. Stretches hips, ankles, and thighs.

2. Relieves neck and lower back pain.

3. Relieves stress by calming down the brain.

Prayer Squat

WHAT TO DO:

1. Adopt a squatting position as in the photo.

2. Place your arm across your chest in prayer position.

3. Breathe diaphragmatically and hold the prayer position for 10 to 60 seconds.

4. As tolerated, use your arms to press your legs apart

5. Focus on releasing your pelvic floor muscles.

WHAT TO WATCH OUT FOR:

1. This can be a very stressful position for women who lack flexibility in the hips and calves.

2. To make the Prayer Pose easier, put some pillows under your feet. You can also do the Prayer Pose against the wall for back support. It might also be helpful to place a pillow underneath the buttocks to take pressure off the body and to make the Prayer Pose easier to handle.

BENEFITS:

1. Opens up the hips, leg and calf muscles.

2 Stretches the calf, back and hip muscles. Because the PFMs are naturally relaxed in this position, it is a great position to use during painful flare-ups.

3. Relieves back pain and hip pain.

You have now been introduced to two of the pillars of your program's foundation, the strengthening and stretching series. Now let's be sure to cover our bases while at the workplace, where we will spend about 40 percent of our time during the weekdays.

Chapter Seven

"When one door closes another door opens;
but we so often look so long and so regretfully
upon the closed door, that we do not see
the ones which open up for us."
— *Alexander Graham Bell*

Chapter 7

STRETCHING AT THE WORKPLACE

I always remember as a child being told that sitting up straight was something very important for me to do. My second-grade teacher would give gold stars to the children who sat upright and tall in their chairs and even a small gift to the child who collected the most stars. This positive reinforcement has remained instilled in me to this day and is a concept that has absolute relevance for my current line of work in treating pelvic pain. Most women with pelvic pain have postural issues as a contributing factor because certain muscles have become inflexible and weak, leading to poor sitting, standing, and walking posture. Sometimes poor posture comes about as a protective mechanism, as women draw inward into their bodies in response to pain and feelings of hopelessness. Women who tell me they want to shut off from the world because their pain has overtaken their lives often assume postures that are hunched over or slouched. Good posture is one of the keys to starting on the road of taking control over your pain. The mind will begin to follow the body if you correct the way you carry yourself. With correct posture you will feel better, think better, and become more confident and reassured about yourself.

The women I treat often sit with poor posture between 6 to 10 hours a day while on the job. By the end of their workday, they complain about various pains and discomforts in the vulva, rectal area, hips, and low back. They find that sitting for any period of time is unbearable, and many grow to dread their jobs for this reason. They report feeling a deep burning sensation from constant pressure on the perineum, a deep ache in their vaginas, or general pain and aches in the hips. They say getting through their workday is sometimes impossible, and many call in sick during their flare-ups, missing workdays and even missing pay.

In these cases, I try to build up their sitting tolerance and give them stretches and pain-relieving strategies they can do at their job. Since bad workplace posture is so prevalent amongst my patients, I have included discreet pain relieving and stress-reducing techniques in *Ending Female Pain*. The stretches can be performed throughout the day. The longer your workday is, the more frequently you should do them. For a typical 8-hour day you should perform the stretches at least 1 to 3 times. Of course if you do these stretches constantly throughout your workday you will achieve greater flexibility, less muscular tension and less sitting pain. Being mindful of your posture can also subliminally contribute to giving you a positive attitude, as you hold your body strong and let your mind know you are not giving up.

Besides the stretches highlighted in this chapter it is extremely important to have your computer workstation set up properly following ergonomic principles. When a patient comes to see me I always ask one critical thing, "What type of job do you do?" This question is key because a poor work environment can be a contributing factor or even a root cause of pain. I also ask, "Has your station been evaluated for proper ergonomics?" The answer from most patients is no. Day after day of bad posture at work contributes to excess strain and stress on the lower back, the pelvic floor muscles, hip muscles, and gluteal muscles.

Many corporate environments have a specialist on staff that will evaluate and correct your workstation environment. If you have a resource like this at your job, use it. Otherwise follow the basic guidelines recommended in this book to check your own work area. There are four areas of focus for a proper set-up: the monitor, the chair, the mouse and the lighting. To set up your computer station correctly and to maintain a healthier work environment make sure your work area adheres to the recommendations listed in Table 7.1. From my personal experience, making the smallest adjustment to your desk environment can make a huge difference to your posture and improve your level of comfort while sitting.

Table: 7.1: Suggestions for a Healthier Work Environment and Proper Computer Ergonomics

WORK CONSIDERATIONS TO REDUCE PELVIC PAIN
1. Position your monitor directly in front of you. You should be able to comfortably view the screen without having to tilt your neck backwards or forwards. A good rule of thumb is that the top of your monitor should be aligned with your forehead and your eyes level to the screen.
2. Your back should be completely supported and straight. Avoid slumping and slouching to prevent straining the lower back and hip muscles. It is essential that you purchase a lumbar roll if your chair does not provide lumbar support. A lumbar roll will help maintain a neutral spine.
3. Make sure to keep your feet flat on the floor. Use a foot stool if necessary. Your upper thighs should be parallel to the floor. Avoid crossing your legs under the chair.
4. Keep elbows at right angles with forearms parallel to the floor. Also keep wrist in a neutral, or flat and straight position.
5. Never hold the phone between your head and shoulder. Use head phones to avoid putting excessive stress on the neck and upper back muscles.
6. Avoid overreaching for the mouse. Your mouse should be near your keyboard.
7. Purchase a good chair. The proper chair has a backrest that can be adjusted. It's best to have the back of the chair incline slightly backwards. This has the effect of relaxing the spinal musculature and decreasing spinal pressure. You can also choose to have the back rest directly upright.
8. Avoid having the monitor too close to your eyes. Recommended distance is from 20 to 25 inches.
9. Avoid storing work-related materials and files below your desk and workstation which can lead to excessive bending, putting unnecessary stress on the back and hip muscles.
10. Take frequent breaks, at least 5 to 10 minutes every hour. While on your breaks do your stretches and releasing exercises.

Now that your computer and work area are optimally aligned and safe for good posture, you need to pay attention to your sitting posture while at your workstation. Correct sitting posture is easy. What's hard for most individuals is to stay within that posture throughout their workday. It is easy to sit in a slumped, forward-head position, but this only contributes to more muscular weakness and pain. For optimal sitting posture follow the recommendations listed in Table 7.2.

Table 7.2: Optimal Sitting Posture for Work and for Exercising on the Job

SPECIAL POSTURE CONSIDERATIONS AT THE WORKPLACE
1. When sitting, maintain a neutral spine at all times. Keep your back straight, knees bent, and head centered over your shoulders. Avoid slouching even though it may feel good at the time. Slouching eventually overstretches spinal ligaments and muscles, creating a vicious cycle oftentimes causing pain.
2. Avoid hiking up or rounding your shoulders while sitting. Shoulders should be relaxed and should drape flat over your ribs.
3. Sit back into the chair so your back is totally supported. Avoid sitting at the front of your chair where you may end up slouching.
4. Your pelvis should be neutral. Avoid rounding the lower back while you are sitting, which adversely affects the nerves that innervate the pelvic muscles and creates excessive stress on your hips and PFM.
5. Don't let your jaw stick out. Align your head with your shoulders and pelvis, and tuck in your chin.
6. Take frequent breaks and avoid sitting for longer than 45 minutes at a time.
7. Keep your feet flat on the floor. Get a stool if needed.

My patients tell me they love their work stretches. They say that their pain is much less at the end of the day; they function better and are able to control pain levels while at work more easily. The following work stretches should be performed at least 1 to 3 times daily or more if needed. All stretches are to be performed in a pain-free range and done only until you feel a gentle stretch in the muscles. Make sure to read the general guidelines found in Table 7.3 and to apply them to all of the stretches in the series.

Table 7.3: Seated Stretch General Guidelines

SPECIAL POSTURE CONSIDERATIONS AT THE WORKPLACE
1. Always use Tension Releasing Breathing, or TRB, while holding stretches. Never hold your breath.
2. Never bounce while holding a stretch.
3. Hold the stretch for as long as tolerated, usually anywhere from 10 seconds to 1 minute.
4. Many of the stretches require that you sit at the front edge of the chair. Always use correct seated posture as described above when not doing the stretch.
5. Always pay attention to your pelvic floor muscles and avoid holding tension in them as you stretch.

Herrera Workplace Stretching Series for Pelvic Pain

Table 7.4: Workplace Stretching Series for Pelvic Pain

Frequency –Monday to Friday

NAME OF STRETCH
1. Seated Half-Wind
2. Seated Side Stretch
3. Seated 4 Stretch
4. Seated Spinal Twist
5. Seated Thigh Release
6. Seated Reverse Kegels
7. Seated Chest Opener
8. Seated Diaphragmatic Breathing

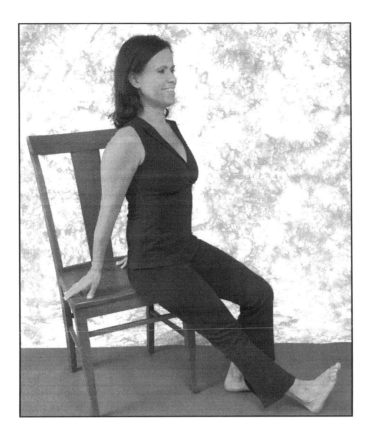

Seated Half-Wind

WHAT TO DO:

   1. Adopt a good seated posture at the edge of your seat.

   2. Straighten out your right leg and point your toes towards your head until you feel a stretch behind the back of your leg and calf.

   3. For deeper stretching, bend forward from the hips while keeping your back straight and shoulders square.

   4. Switch legs and repeat.

WHAT TO WATCH OUT FOR:

1. Watch out for pain radiating into the toes. If this occurs, stretch less aggressively, keeping the foot in a more neutral position instead of pointing it up. Stop immediately if pain persists despite modification.

2. If you experience pain or discomfort in the lower back, make sure you remain upright instead of leaning forward. If pain continues in the lower back muscles, stop.

3. Poor postural alignment while doing this stretch can put excessive strain on your upper and lower back muscles. Make sure you don't overarch your back as well.

BENEFITS:

1. This stretch improves hamstring and calf flexibility.

2. Relieves tension in pelvic floor muscles via fascial connections throughout the hamstrings.

3. Helps to decrease lower back pain encouraging good posture and pelvic/ hip alignment.

Seated Side Stretch

WHAT TO DO:

1. Start in a seated position at the front of your chair, using good posture as outlined earlier in the chapter.

2. Raise your right arm up towards ceiling and place your left arm at your hips.

3. Bend your upper body to the left while reaching up and over with your right arm.

4. Bring your body back to the center and repeat the pose on the other side.

WHAT TO WATCH OUT FOR:

1. Avoid compressing into the left side. Think tall as you bend sideways.

2. Avoid overstretching and forcing the side-bend as this can cause pain to the intercostals or side muscles.

BENEFITS:

1. Helps increase the flexibility of your spine, arms, and rib cage.

2. Helps to realign pelvic bones and maintain lumbar spine and sacral alignment.

3. Enhances nerve function.

4. Facilitates rib expansion which will help get more oxygen into your lungs and promote better breathing.

Seated 4 Stretch

WHAT TO DO:

1. While seated in good posture at the edge of your seat, place the left ankle lightly on the thigh of the right leg making a figure 4. Keep your hips square, your shoulders down and back as you sit straight.

2. If you are able, gently press your crossed leg down but not lower than your thigh.

3. For a deeper stretch, lean forward from the hips with a straight back. For an even deeper stretch rotate your upper body slightly towards your feet.

4. Bring your body back to center and repeat the pose on the other side.

WHAT TO WATCH OUT FOR:

1. Don't torque the ankle bone. Remember to keep the ankle bone slightly off the resting thigh to avoid stressing it.

2. Avoid slouching in this posture to prevent stress on the lumbar spinal nerves and to make this stretch more effective.

3. If your pain increases and/or radiates into your thigh or lower leg/foot, or persists for 30 minutes or longer, discontinue this stretch and consult your healthcare professional.

BENEFITS:

1. Helps prevent sciatica.

2. Helps to stretch the piriformis muscle and maintain pelvic alignment.

3. Helps increase the mobility and function of the major nerve roots of the lumbar and sacral spine which innervate the pelvic floor muscles and internal pelvic organs.

4. Improves blood flow to the hip and pelvic muscles.

Seated Spinal Twist

WHAT TO DO:

1. Sit at the edge of your seat and cross your right thigh over your left thigh. Place your left hand on your right knee and gently pull the knee across the body.

2. Place your right hand behind you, open up the chest and lengthen your spine upward, bringing your gaze over your right shoulder while simultaneously twisting.

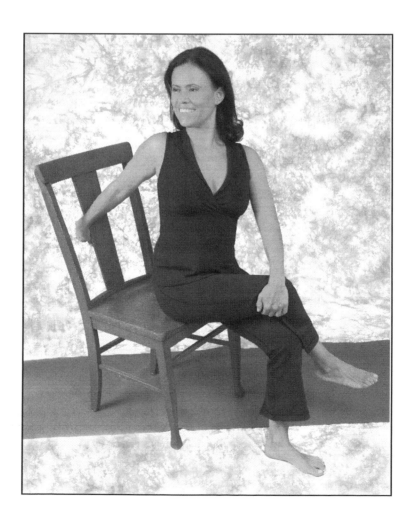

3. Inhale, straighten the spine, and then exhale, twisting gently until you feel a mild stretch in your right hip muscles and back muscles.

WHAT TO WATCH OUT FOR:

1. Avoid overtwisting and straining the back muscles.

2. Make sure you do not slouch and compress the spinal column while twisting. You have to stay tall and straight as you do this exercise.

3. Avoid pulling the knee across the body too vigorously.

BENEFITS:

1. Increases nourishment to the roots of the spinal nerves and the sympathetic nervous system.

2. Improves flexibility throughout the spinal column and also helps to mobilize the vertebrae.

3. Cleanses the body. Do it the day after overindulging with food and drink.

Seated Thigh Release

WHAT TO DO:

    1. Sit at the edge of your seat in good posture, with your back straight and chin tucked.

    2. Gently widen your legs until a stretch is felt in the inner thigh muscles.

    3. For a deeper stretch, place hands on inner thigh muscles and press them gently outwards.

WHAT TO WATCH OUT FOR:

    1. Avoid poor postural alignment and rounding of the lower back.

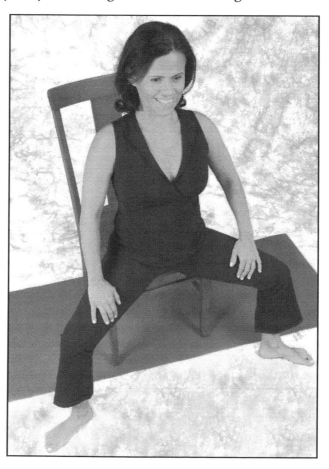

2. Do not apply too much pressure on the thighs as this can cause micro-tears in the inner thigh muscles.

BENEFITS:

1. Increases flexibility of the inner thigh, also called adductor muscles.

2. Helps to decrease trigger points in the inner thigh muscles which are quite common in women with pelvic pain.

3. Indirectly stretches out the perineum and brings blood flow to the area which is often blocked after hours of sitting.

Seated Chest Opener

WHAT TO DO:

1. Sit with good posture on the edge of your seat.

2. Clasp your hands behind your back, interlocking your fingers.

3. Roll your shoulders down and back, stretching your chest upward.

4. Raise your arms slightly upward, tucking your chin under.

WHAT TO WATCH OUT FOR:

1. Don't stick out your chin as this puts pressure on your neck.

2. Don't slouch in this pose. Sit up straight.

BENEFITS:

1. Improves posture.

2. Decreases upper and lower back pain.

3. Psychologically opens you up and puts you in a position of confidence.

Seated Reverse Kegels (Read Chapter 4 for more details)
WHAT TO DO:

1. Sit with good posture on the front of your chair with your weight evenly distributed on your sit bones.

2. Place your right hand on your right sit bone, your left hand on left sit bone, with palms facing up.

3. With your mind's eye and Tension Releasing Breath (TRB), direct your inhalation breath to your PFMs for 5 seconds, while simultaneously visualizing that your sit bones are moving apart and your pelvic floor muscles are releasing and dropping into the chair.

4. This is a very difficult exercise to do. As you get better at releasing the tension in your PFMs, you will no longer have to place your hands on your sit bones. You will be able to let go of tension in your pelvic floor in any position and at any time.

WHAT TO WATCH OUT FOR:

Avoid holding the breath and pushing out the PFMs.

BENEFITS:

Releases tension and creates flexibility in the PFMs.

Seated Diaphragmatic Breathing

WHAT TO DO:

1. Sit with good posture and place one hand on your chest and the other over your belly button.

2. Focus on your breathing. Breathe in deeply, expanding the belly outward and keeping the chest from moving too much. Then exhale with pursed lips to control the release of air, trying to keep the inhale and the exhale at the same number of seconds.

3. When you inhale, think of the word *stress* and when you exhale, think of the word *free*.

4. Focus on releasing your PFMs while doing this technique.

WHAT TO WATCH OUT FOR:

1. Do not allow thoughts besides the words *stress* and *free* to enter your mind. If this occurs, say the word *thinking* and return to the words *stress* and *free*.

2. Avoid taking in too much air at once or holding your breath. Keep your breathing smooth.

3. Don't breathe with excessive chest and neck movements, which is the opposite of diaphragmatic breathing. Non-diaphragmatic breathing is ineffective in relieving stress and clearing the mind.

BENEFITS:

1. Reduces stress and anxiety. Women with stressful jobs or those experiencing flare-ups will benefit from practicing diaphragmatic breathing at work for 10 to 20 breaths every hour on the hour.

2. Helps with pain control.

3. Allows more oxygen to enter the lungs.

4. Facilitates healing by increasing proper diaphragmatic movement and excursion of the ribs. It's important to remember that the major vessels that bring blood to the pelvic and abdominal areas travel through the diaphragm. So if the diaphragm is not moving properly, blood flow is compromised to the pelvic and abdominal organs and muscles.

We have covered a lot of ground already, laying out the key concepts for our foundation, strengthening with Kegels, stretching, and what to do at work. Now let's add the final component to our foundation, which is the foam roller series, so we can learn to release muscle pain and trigger points before they become a chronic problem.

Chapter Eight

*"Always bear in mind that
your own resolution to succeed is
more important than any other thing."*
—Abraham Lincoln

Chapter 8

FOAM ROLLER MYOFASCIAL-MASSAGE AND RELEASE TECHNIQUES

Myofascial pain is a phrase that many of us are hearing more about today. Myofascial pain can be described as pain, trigger points or spasms, or sensitive areas found between muscles and fascia. Everyone knows what muscles are but fascia is a little bit more esoteric. Imagine the human body without muscles, bones, blood and fat. What would be left is a skeletal form that looks like a human body but is made of connective tissue. Fascia is a complex network of connective tissue that surrounds everything in the human body.

Many of the women I treat who suffer from pelvic conditions have moderate to severe myofascial restrictions in the muscles that attach to the pelvis and to the pelvic floor muscles. These restrictions can be classified as spasms, adhesions, knots and painful trigger points. To release these restricted muscular areas I teach all my patients to use my foam roller release series which I have included in this book.

With a foam roller you can give yourself a deep tissue massage without the hefty price tag. It's probably not as effective as a hands-on massage; however, you can do your foam rolling anywhere, anytime, and with practice your body will feel less painful, longer, softer and more flexible.

The foam roller works via the Golgi Tendon Organ (GTO) found in the area where muscles and tendon are. The GTO responds to changes in muscular tension. When you increase the pressure and/or tension in the muscles to the point where the muscle is overstrained, the GTO responds by relaxing the muscle. This is called autogenic inhibition. By exciting the GTO, muscles and fascia surrounding the muscles are able to relax helping to increase flexibility and range of motion and decreasing pain naturally.

The foam roller massage is one of my favorite self-treatment tools that uses your own body weight to release myofascial pain and trigger points found in muscles. The foam roller is tube-shaped Styrofoam that varies in shape, density and hardness. It's an inexpensive piece of equipment that is a necessary tool for women to combat conditions that afflict the pelvic floor. As you roll over your muscles, you release fascial restrictions as well as muscular trigger points and muscles spasms which restrict blood flow and do not allow your body to get rid of toxins. The foam roller also helps to soften scar tissue and muscular adhesions below surgical sites.

Many of the women I treat love their foam roller exercises and tell me they feel their muscles become softer, their pain decrease and their stress diminish. The object is to find the restrictions in muscles which tend to be hard, painful areas and to roll the painful areas slowly and deliberately for a minimum of 2 minutes until the pain decreases by at least 50 percent. Once you find a painful spot, you can also rock over the areas from side to side to increase the release of the muscle. Use the foam roller as a tool to get to know your body. You will be amazed at how many areas you will find in parts of your body that you have not thought about before. Before getting started, please read through the following charts which highlight the benefits, precautions and recommendations to consider before undertaking the foam roller series.

Table 8.1: What to Watch Out for While Performing the Foam Rolling Series

PRECAUTION
1. Avoid rolling over bony areas.
2. Avoid rolling over open wounds.
3. Avoid rolling over young, acute injuries.
4. Avoid rolling over abdominal scar younger than 6 weeks unless you get clearance from your surgeon.
5. Expect to have some muscle soreness after the rolling. If you have excessive soreness, wait 24 to 36 hours before rolling that body part again.
6. If you have circulatory problems, discuss with your doctor before starting the foam rolling exercises.
7. Avoid rolling over the abdominal area if you are experiencing moderate to severe menstrual cramps.

Table 8.2: Benefits of Self-Myofascial and Trigger Point Release with Foam Rollers

BENEFIT
1. Helps to maintain normal muscle length.
2. Improves muscle flexibility.
3. Decreases lactic acid build-up.
4. Decreases muscles adhesions and reduces scar tissue.
5. Helps eliminate trigger points, spasms and painful knots.
6. Helps increase muscle range of motion.
7. Helps to correct muscular imbalances.
8. Decreases excessive tone of muscles creating suppleness in the muscles.
9. Helps improve blood flow to muscles.
10. Releases toxins from muscles.
11. Helps reduce stress and anxiety in the body and mind.

Table 8.3: Foam Rolling Myofascial and Trigger Point Release Series

FOAM ROLLER POSITION
1. Foam Roller Upper Back Release
2. Foam Roller Sacral Rolling
3. Foam Roller Lower Back Rolling
4. Foam Roller Rolling Front of Thighs
5. Foam Roller Inner Thigh/Groin
6. Foam Roller Piriformis and Gluteal Muscle Release
7. Foam Roller Side Hip Roll - Iliotibial Band (ITB)
8. Foam Roller Quadratus Lumborum (QL) Release
9. Foam Roller Goddess
10. Foam Roller Abdominal Muscle and Scar Rolling
11. Foam Roller Sacrotuberus-Upper Hamstring

Table 8.4: Foam Rolling Recommendations

GUIDELINE
1. Drink plenty of fluids after your foam rolling sessions.
2. Roll each muscle for 1 to 3 minutes or as tolerated.
3. Keep your back straight when necessary and avoid sagging the lower back to avoid injury.
4. When rolling over painful areas or muscular knots and trigger points, roll more slowly and with shorter rolls over the painful area until you feel a muscular release or the pain starts to diminish by 50 percent. This reduction in pain may take longer than 2 minutes.
5. In additional to rolling along the body part, remember to also rock back and forth sideways with short strokes to get deeper into the trigger points and spasms you uncover.
6. For painful trigger points, keep the pressure for at least 90 seconds. Repeat as necessary until the pain decreases by 50 percent or more.
7. To reduce the effects of gravity on the body, reduce pressure and decrease pain over a muscle, do one of the following: • Keep both legs on the foam roller. • Avoid stacking the legs over each other. • Support your body as much as possible by keeping hands, feet and elbows on the floor.
8. Avoid sagging into the shoulder joint when rolling on hands. Shoulders have to be away from the ears and chest should be lifted.
9. Breathe diaphragmatically and also use Tension Releasing Breathing or TRB (see chapter 6, page 102) while rolling. Do not hold your breath while performing foam roller exercises
10. Pay close attention to your pelvic floor muscles. Keep them relaxed as you roll over them.
11. Focus on the problem areas first until you get relief. Foam rolling can be performed everyday.

Foam Rolling Myofascial and Trigger Point Release Series
Foam Roller Upper Back Release

WHAT TO DO:

1. Place foam roller on your mid-back with your hands behind your head.

2. For neck support, keep your knees bent with your feet close to the buttocks.

3. Gently roll up and down on the thoracic spine and mid-back muscles.

4. Avoid pulling and/or hyperextending your neck.

5. Roll 1 to 2 minutes over your mid-back muscles. Focus on the painful spots and concentrate the rolling and rocking on those areas that cause you the most pain.

6. For trigger points, stay on the spots, applying consistent pressure over them for 90 seconds.

7. For muscle spasms, apply consistent pressure and do little clockwise or counterclockwise circles until pain subsides.

Foam Roller Sacral Rolling

WHAT TO DO:

1. Balance on the foam roller with both hands behind you on the floor, placing your sacrum on the foam roller.

2. Keep your hands close to the foam roller to avoid straining your shoulders.

3. Without collapsing your shoulders, gently roll up and down on the sacrum. Remember to maintain good upright posture with the chest lifted.

4. Roll 1 to 2 minutes over your sacrum. Focus on the painful spots and concentrate the rolling and rocking on that area.

Foam Roller Lower Back Rolling

WHAT TO DO:

1. Place the foam roller on your lower back and balance on your hands behind you. Keep your hands close to the foam roller to avoid straining your shoulders.

2. Without collapsing the chest and shoulders, gently roll up and down the lower back muscles. Remember to maintain good upright posture with the chest lifted.

3. Roll 1 to 2 minutes over your lower back muscles. Focus on the painful spots and concentrate the rolling and rocking on that area.

Foam Roller Rolling Front of Thighs

WHAT TO DO:

1. Balance on your elbows and place the foam roller on the front of your thighs. Keeping your abdominals slightly engaged and your back straight, roll from the upper knee to the top of the thighs. Avoid going over the kneecaps.

2. Roll 1 to 2 minutes over your thighs. Focus on the painful spots and concentrate the rolling and rocking on the areas where you find pain and restrictions.

Foam Roller Inner Thigh/Groin

WHAT TO DO:

1. Balance on your elbows and place the foam roller on the right inner thigh by flexing the right hip to the side and bending the knee. You may have to move your hands for better rolling. Your elbows should both be on one side of the roller.

2. Slowly roll from the top of the groin to the knee.

3. Break up the rolling into the upper groin, the middle inner thigh and the lower thigh area for better emphasis. Avoid rolling over the knee joint.

4. Roll 1 to 2 minutes over your inner thighs. Focus on the painful spots and concentrate the rolling and rocking on the areas where you find pain and restrictions.

5. Switch legs and repeat on the other side.

Foam Roller Piriformis and Gluteal Muscle Release

WHAT TO DO:

1. Place the foam roller on the right buttock cheek with the ankle of the left foot across your right thigh.

2. Balancing on the right hand and right foot, slowly roll the gluteal and piriformis muscles from top to bottom. Keep your left arm balanced on the left knee.

3. Avoid collapsing the shoulders.

4. Roll 1 to 2 minutes over your gluteal and piriformis muscles. Focus on the painful spots and concentrate the rolling on that area.

5. Repeat on the other leg.

Foam Roller Side Hip Roll – Iliotibial Band (ITB)

WHAT TO DO:

1. Place the foam roller at the top of the hip bone and balance on your elbows as shown in the photo. You can also balance on the right hand if you have difficulty balancing on your elbow.

2. Keeping the body perpendicular to the foam roller, slowly roll up and down the side of the hip. Focus on the hot spots or painful spots as you roll up and down.

3. Roll 1 to 2 minutes over your ITB. Focus on the painful spots and concentrate the rolling on that area. If too painful to roll the full length of the ITB, break up the rolling into upper ITB, middle ITB, and lower ITB.

Foam Roller Quadratus Lumborum (QL) Release

WHAT TO DO:

1. Place the foam roller on the right side of the body between the rib and hip bone.

2. Balance on your right elbow and your right foot and bend your right leg in front of you.

3. Make sure you do not roll over your ribs with this exercise as you could actually break a bone if you roll over your ribs.

4. Roll 1 to 2 minutes over your quadratus lumborum (QL) muscles. Focus on the painful spots and concentrate the rolling on that area.

Foam Roller Goddess

WHAT TO DO:

1. Lie on the foam roller with outstretched hands. Make sure to keep your entire spine on the foam roller as you practice your diaphragmatic breathing.

2. Visualize the stress leaving your body as you focus on areas of the spine that feel tight.

3. Practice your diaphragmatic breathing or mind body techniques for 5 minutes or longer.

Foam Roller Abdominal Muscle and Scar Rolling

WHAT TO DO:

1. Balance on your elbows and place the foam roller on the abdominals. Roll from the bottom of the abdominals to the top. If you have abdominal scars, do abdominal rolls on it to release any fascial restrictions.

Foam Roller Sacrotuberous-Upper Hamstring

WHAT TO DO:

1. Sit high on your sit bones with legs in front of you. Make sure to maintain good, straight posture. Keeping your abdominals slightly engaged, roll gently back and forth on your sit bones.

2. Roll from the top of the sit bones to the top of the hamstring insertion, or upper back of the thighs. Focus on the hot spots and do small rolls. Be sure to avoid slumping the lower back.

Now that our foundation is set, let's build a second layer on top in which we will directly access our own pelvic floor muscles with internal and external techniques. One of the most important aspects of your self-healing journey is to work directly on your pelvic floor muscles (PFMs). How do you do this? By accessing the muscles directly, through a variety of internal and external techniques that are outlined in Part III. Remember, think of your PFM spasms and trigger points as similar to those that some people get in their shoulders and neck muscles. Your pelvic floor muscles, like any other muscles, are susceptible to the same kinds of injuries. They can be treated in the same way we treat other body spasms, with myofascial and trigger point release, scar adhesion release, massage, and stretching.

If you approach your pelvic floor muscle or scar pain like any other muscle pain in your body, you can quickly get over your fears of doing the detective work in these sensitive areas and find the painful spots in your body. You must scientifically construct your internal and external release series with the tools in this section of the book.

Unlike the yoga, Pilates ball, and foam roller series, there is no set order for these techniques. I have laid out a toolbox for you to try, based on the tried and true techniques that I teach my patients to incorporate into their daily routines. If you find yourself hitting roadblocks or not making progress, consider seeking the help of a physical therapist that specializes in PFM work to get you on the right track. Also make sure to read the precautions in each chapter of Part III before starting your PFM release or scar program. If you are suffering from any of the symptoms listed, consult your medical doctor before you begin these techniques.

Most importantly, you must listen to what your body is saying. I firmly believe that everyone holds the key to her own healing, which is why I have written this book. Some of the techniques may elicit more pain in the short term but end up being very effective over time. When used in combination with your Kegel, breathing, yoga stretching, and Pilates ball strengthening programs, these powerful techniques can supercharge your pain relief.

Remember to use the pain mapping recommendations from Chapter 3 to really get a good sense of your body's trigger points and spasms. With a bit of grit and determination you can begin to get on the right path to reducing your painful symptoms. I cannot stress enough that you may experience an increase of your symptoms for 24 to 72 hours after you do your internal work. This is normal. Just rest, continue your reverse Kegel and stretching techniques, and resume the internal work once you feel better. The techniques in the next chapters of this book are designed to decrease hypertonicity, improve mobility, decrease pain, eliminate trigger points and improve everyday function.

In Their Own Words – Doctor to Doctor without Answers

"I had been suffering with pelvic pain for 4 months before I started physical therapy. I had been to a handful of doctors, most of whom were baffled by my condition. I had never had pelvic pain before - one day I just woke up with terrible itching and burning, and sex had become incredibly painful. I arrived at physical therapy with little hope of recovery - I had basically resigned myself to a lifetime of painful sex and discomfort (it was a regular occurrence for me to shed a few tears during my first few weeks of therapy). However, once I started a regimen (and started thinking positively), I began to see results and experience some relief. It took dedication and perseverence - physical therapy can be time consuming and sometimes painful, but I continued on day after day with the hope that one day my pain would go away. It has been about a year since the onset of my pelvic pain, and I am now almost completely pain and itch free. I have even been able to wean myself off of the medications I was on (which my doctor had prescribed to help with pelvic muscle spasms), which I never thought possible. Before the onset of my condition, I had never heard of physical therapy for pelvic pain, but I am so lucky and grateful to have found people like the therapists at Renew PT who understood my condition and helped me to recover."

Part 3
Self-Care Techniques for the Pelvic Floor

"Happiness is not something ready made.
It comes from your own actions."
— *Dalai Lama*

Chapter 9

DECREASING PELVIC FLOOR MUSCLE PAIN WITH INTERNAL DILATOR STRETCHES AND INTERNAL HANDS-ON TECHNIQUES

The internal techniques listed in this chapter are designed to be done with dilators or your fingers. Sometimes you may find it difficult to reach certain muscles with your fingers and will have to use your dilators. If you find yourself feeling uneasy about using dilators in general, give it some time and start slow. With practice, you will reap the benefits of these powerful techniques.

Table 9.1: Precautions to Consider Before Starting Internal Hands-On Techniques

Get clearance from your doctor before starting vaginal or abdominal techniques outlined in this chapter, IF YOU:
1. Have just had surgery.
2. Have just given birth and have a scar from an episiotomy, perineal tear or perineal repair.
3. Have a vaginal or abdominal scar infection or bleeding.
4. Have just given birth. Wait six weeks before massaging perineal scars and only if you get clearance from your doctor.
5. Experience any increase in scar pain. Get checked to make sure the scar is healing well.
If you have started on the techniques but experience any of the following, STOP:
1. If you feel tingling down the leg or in the perineum. Stop and get off the spot as you are probably on a nerve.

2. If you feel numbness down the leg or in the perineum. Stop and get off the spot as you are probably on an artery.

3. If you smell a foul odor coming from your vagina, abdominal or perineal scar. This could be a sign of infection and must be reported to your caregiver.

4. If you get on a spot that has a pulse. You are probably on an artery and want to avoid compressing into the blood supply.

General Guidelines:

1. Avoid massaging and pressing the tendinous arch of the levator ani muscles. This tendon feels like a cooked spaghetti noodle and is usually very painful to touch. See Diagram 3.1 on page 31 for the location of this tendon.

2. You may be able to massage more vigorously if you have had an internal Botox injection to relax your PFMs.

Dilators

A great way to eliminate painful trigger points and to get your PFMs supple and pain-free again is to do daily dilator stretches. At first many of my patients feel strange about doing this kind of exercise, in such a personal area, with a thing that looks like a small dildo. Many of you will also have fear and anxiety having to look at and touch your vaginas. Just like you would stretch your hamstrings on a daily basis, stretching your vaginal muscles is a normal and necessary thing to do if you are suffering from conditions like painful sex or muscle spasms. Look at stretching your vaginal muscles with a dilator not in a sexual context but as a medical necessity that will help you regain a pain-free life. For many of you, you will not achieve pain-free sex unless you incorporate intra-vaginal stretching on a daily basis into your exercise program. This type of therapy is an integral part of your sexual healing.

Dilators are healing devices that will assist you in stretching out your PFMs and reducing pain associated with sex and activities of daily living. Many women have pain during intercourse, and the dilator is a great tool that helps open up and release this area. Dilators are also great for relieving deep trigger points found in the inner layers of the PFMs.

Dilators come in different graduated sizes. Most of my patients start with extra small and gradually move up as their muscles become stretched, less painful, and open. These different sizes help to stretch the vaginal muscles so that sexual penetration is not painful. Some of my patients who had experienced intense pain with penetration but who have now graduated to the largest dilator, still fear having sexual relations even though their muscles are stretched out and pain-free. With practice, dilators can help you overcome your fear of penetration.

Crystal Wand

Another tool that is a great resource is called the Crystal Wand. This curved device can be used for hard to reach spots in the innermost layers of the pelvic floor.

To reduce any anxiety you might have before starting the PFM stretching, become familiar with your dilator before your session. Feel the dilator's hard smooth texture, press it against your body and examine the different sizes in your set, if you already have more than one. Another great way to prepare yourself for this type of stretching is to meditate for 5 to 10 minutes before you begin your session, incorporating diaphragmatic breathing to release tension and reduce anxiety. I find that many of my patients also try to see the humor in their situation and find that giving the dilator a name keeps the internal work lighter and less emotionally charged.

Dilator sizes vary in their diameter, getting progressively wider. Some dilator sets come with 4 different sizes, and others up to 8. The set that I use with my patients has 4 dilators to a set, and I number them 1 to 4, from smallest to largest (see photo on page 161). To use them correctly, make sure you have a basic knowledge of your vaginal anatomy and muscles as I have defined in Chapter 3 of the book. I also find that when my patients are consistent with their exercises they experience less pain with sex, sitting, positional changes and standing, and are ultimately happier.

In Their Own Words – One Patient's Pre- and Post-Surgical Story

"I noticed the first symptoms of vestibulodynia (VVS) about six months after my wedding. For a while, I had been treated with strong antibiotics for a persistent stomach parasite, and each of the 3 courses of antibiotics had left me with bad yeast infections. These yeast infections never seemed to go away even though I eventually found a doctor who gave me daily oral antifungals. During this time, I avoided sex because sex with a yeast infection is a pretty bad idea. It hurts and you can pass it back and forth between partners. Even when I finally tested negative for yeast, the pain was still there. In fact, it was more intense than before. On penetration, I felt a tearing, burning sensation that temporarily disappeared but returned more intensely after sex. It felt like I was on fire, it was unbearable. For as long as 48 hours after sex, I was plagued by burning, itching and stabbing sensations in my vestibular area. It felt like having a UTI each time I had sex.

"My doctor said she believed it was vestibulodynia and suggested I try a steroid cream. In Australia (where I was living at that time), they tend to be more conservative in their medical approach. While this is often a good thing, I think a more aggressive treatment at the outset yields a better outcome for vestibulodynia. Steroid cream was commonly prescribed 5 years ago, but it is rarely done today because it has been known to further weaken the skin of the vulva, making it even more prone to tearing. After a few months she referred me to a gynecologist, who was very kind and understanding. She put me back on daily oral antifungals and prescribed physical therapy. I had 2 sessions with the therapists before being discharged, but I did not get any better. I tried a low-oxalate diet, which did nothing but make me skeletally thin. Then I saw an acupuncturist who may have helped my sinuses, but did nothing for my VVS.

"In 2004, I moved back to New York and decided to consult a pioneering doctor in Boston who was amazing. She listened to my history and treated the condition very aggressively. Over the course of the next 2 years, I had some improvement, mostly from lidocaine cream. Unfortunately, I just didn't respond well enough and it became clear that I would be one of the very rare cases for whom surgery was going to be the best option. In 2006, my doctor referred me to Isa Herrera at Renew PT to begin physical therapy in preparation for my surgery. I had a very dim view of physical therapy based on my experiences in Sydney. But Isa proved to be my secret weapon against VVS. She has made it her life's work to understand how to unlock the body to lessen the grip of vaginal pain. Isa got me ready both physically and psychologically to face the frightening realities of a vestibulectomy. Whenever I would get discouraged, she would help me build up my mental framework and shore me up against the frustrations of this very mentally-challenging disease.

"I would like to use this space to talk a little about the surgery itself. I don't think doctors are entirely clear about how big an impact this surgery has on your body and mind. Maybe they don't want you to build it up and be afraid or maybe they just don't get it. But I feel that having all the information at hand would have been better, so I will relate my experience here.

"A vestibulectomy is not a small surgery. It is not a 'glorified episiotomy' as I have heard it called. The surgery I had, which in all fairness was more radical than average, was brutal. I bled far longer than the aftercare sheet said I would. I was unable to leave Boston after the surgery because my bleeding was so heavy the doctor wanted me to stay near the hospital to be on the safe side. I was in ridiculously searing pain for the first ten days or so. And even once the nightmare was over, there was the plain fact that I was physically too small for even a routine pap smear with a speculum. Isa helped me stretch out the vaginal opening with dilators, which are basically just medical-grade dildos, over the course of a long, long time. My recovery period from surgery to pain-free sex took 8 months. But then again, you may have caught that last bit: pain-free sex. Yes, the surgery is horrible and the recovery is only slightly less so, but I am 95 percent better. No more burning and itching after sex. Next month will mark one year since the surgery and thanks to my doctor in Boston and the fantastic care at Renew PT, I can wear tight jeans, ride a bike, and have sex like a newlywed."

Getting Started

To start, you should have a mirror, pillows, vaginal lubricant, and if you like, non-latex gloves. For vaginal lubricants I like to use FireFly™, Slippery Wet™ or old-fashioned olive oil, vitamin E oil, or rose oil. Make sure you do not have allergies to any of these products. I am also a big fan of lubricants that are organic and alcohol free, if you have access to any of these products. For organic and hypoallergenic products, visit your local health food store or your local sex shop.

The vaginal stretching exercises can be done in several different positions, but to familiarize yourself with the techniques, starting off in a semi-reclined position with a pillow under your head will work great. If your hip muscles are very tight or if you become uncomfortable, place a pillow under each thigh so that your knees are supported. Later on you can experiment with one leg up supported on the toilet or bench. You can even try lying on your side, which is also a great position.

Table 9.2: Internal Techniques for Pelvic Muscle Release Using a Dilator or Finger

NAME OF TECHNIQUE
1. General Pelvic Floor Muscle Stretching
2. Pelvic Floor Muscle Clock Stretching
3. Pelvic Floor Myofascial Release
4. Internal PFM Trigger Point Release
5. Internal PFM Cross Friction Fiber Massage
6. Internal PFM Half-Moon Strumming Massage

General Pelvic Floor Muscle Stretching
WHAT TO DO:

1. Clean your dilator with hot water and soap. Avoid using antibacterial wipes and antibacterial soaps. Use the same soap that you use to clean your body. I recommend hypoallergenic soap like Aveeno™. Some silicone dilators can be cleaned by placing them in boiling water for a few minutes.

2. To keep the dilator warm, place it in a cup of warm water until you are ready to use it.

3. Apply a generous amount of lubricant to your vaginal opening. Dry off the dilator and place plenty of lubricant on its tip.

4. Practice diaphragmatic breathing for a couple of breaths and do a couple of reverse Kegels or contract/relax Kegels as defined in Part II. This will help relax your PFM before insertion of the dilator, and will make your experience more comfortable. You may also want to do your yoga series before you begin so you can be in a more relaxed state.

5. When you are ready both mentally and physically, slowly insert the dilator into your vaginal opening, angling the dilator downwards towards your tailbone. The dilators are usually 6 to 8 inches long but initially try inserting it 2 to 3 inches. ONLY insert the dilator to your physical and emotional comfort level. The dilator is not meant to go all the way inside; you should be able to hold on to the end of it. Continue inserting it, stopping periodically to practice your diaphragmatic breathing, your reverse Kegel, and your contract/relax Kegels, which will help you insert it deeper.

6. Avoid inserting or pressing the dilator in the 12 o'clock or top position because your bladder is located there and there are no muscles to stretch at this position. Inserting it in this position could also cause bladder pain, or worse, could possibly damage the bladder tissue.

7. At first keep the dilator inside the vagina anywhere from 5 minutes to an hour everyday, depending on how much you can tolerate. When you feel you are ready, you can thrust the dilator in and out to simulate sexual intercourse. Do not do more than you can tolerate. This in-and-out motion can be done at any time during your dilator routine and with any size dilator. The key thing is to make sure you are psychologically and emotionally prepared to do it.

8. Try advancing to the next size dilator after a week or 2 of consistent exercising with the smaller dilator. Do not advance to the next size unless you are comfortable with inserting it, moving it around, and there is little or no pain when using your current dilator.

9. To advance to the next dilator it is sometimes helpful to switch back and forth between dilator sizes for comfort and to get used to the larger size. When you switch between sizes, relubricate and insert slowly especially if going from smaller to bigger. Remember that you will decide how to advance your own dilator stretching program. The key concept to ensure success and to put you on the road to pain-free sex is being consistent with your dilator exercises. If you fall off the wagon with your exercises, start your program again as soon as possible. Remember to always be gentle with yourself and do not let your mind fill with negative self-talk. Be gentle with yourself as you progress because it takes time!

10. Your goal is to be able to fit a dilator comfortably inside your vagina that is one size bigger than your partner's penis.

Pelvic Floor Muscle Clock Stretching

GETTING STARTED:

The pelvic floor muscle clock stretching techniques work great for women who are having trouble getting the dilators into their vaginas, or for those women who have pain with initial penetration, painful scars, or spasms in their muscles. For this method, imagine again that your vaginal opening is a clock.

To review, 12 o'clock is by the clitoris, 6 o'clock is by the rectum, 3 o'clock is to the left and 9 o'clock is to the right. Using your smallest dilator or finger, start stretching your vagina using the clock as visualization. Remember that the PFMs are divided into 3 layers, each layer corresponding to the knuckles of the finger and progressively deeper inside the vagina. The first PFM layer is knuckle 1, the second PFM layer is knuckle 2, and the third PFM layer is knuckle 3.

WHAT TO DO:

Diagram 9.1: Clock

1. Focus your stretching from 3 to 9 o'clock positions avoiding 12 o'clock where the bladder is located.

2. Start with PFM Layer 1, then progress to Layer 2, and then to Layer 3, only when you feel comfortable and confident.

3. Press around the clock for 30 to 60 seconds or until you feel a release in the vaginal muscles. You can go around the clock 2 to 3 times or you can stay on the same spot for 3 repetitions of 30 to 60 seconds.

4. For women who have just had babies or for those who have undergone surgeries, it is best to wait at least 6 weeks and get cleared by your childbirth caregiver before starting your clock stretching program.

5. The main thing is to decrease the pain as you press into the muscles. I always aim for at least 50 percent reduction in pain when I do the clock stretches on my patients.

6. Oils that can be used for stretching are vitamin E oil, rose oil and any lubricant that is organic and alcohol free.

Pelvic Floor Muscle Myofascial Release

GETTING STARTED:

Myofascial stretching and release of the PFMs is one of the best techniques in this chapter to improve mobility, decrease pain, increase strength, and decrease hypertonicity, creating more supple muscles. To visualize the technique, imagine that your PFMs are 3-dimensional, like a tube. There are 3 layers to the tube from superficial to the deepest layer. The tube is further divided with 2 outer walls on the left and right, an inferior wall, near the rectum, and a superior wall, towards the bladder. Now imagine that the walls of the tube described above are now divided in half the long way, a right half and a left half. The left half corresponds to the clock at 1, 2, 3, 4, 5, 6 o'clock, and the right half corresponds to the 6, 7, 8, 9, 10, 11, and 12 o'clock position. This methodology is also helpful for doing advanced pain mapping as well to help you track the location of your pain.

WHAT TO DO:

1. Place some lubricant on your dilator or finger and insert your finger or dilator into the third or deepest layer at the 2 o'clock position. On your finger this corresponds to the third knuckle. This technique requires that you

Diagram 9.2: Cylinder and Clock

Base Image: Netter Images

apply gentle yet firm pressure throughout the PFM layer by layer.

2. Using your dilator or finger apply gentle yet firm pressure for 20 to 30 seconds on the left half of the third layer at 2 o'clock. Repeat for 3, 4, 5, and 6 o'clock positions in the third layer. Then continue on the left side and repeat the 2 to 6 o'clock positions on the second and then first PFM layers.

3. Once you have completed the left half of the myofascial technique, go to the right side and repeat the same 20 to 30 second pressure release at 10, 9, 8, 7, and 6 o'clock positions through the deepest PFM Layer 3 to the superficial PFM Layer 1.

4. You may find very painful spots as you move through the layers and around the clock. If you come across a layer that is extremely painful, you have found a trigger point. Take note of its location and use the trigger point release method that follows to attack and eliminate it.

Internal Pelvic Floor Muscle Trigger Point Release
GETTING STARTED:

Use this method hand-in-hand with the myofascial release technique. Trigger point therapy is not a quick-fix solution for chronic pelvic pain. It can take weeks and even months to stabilize the pain. The one thing that is important to understand is that once you have mastered these basic techniques you will be able to take back control over the pain. To be successful with the trigger point release techniques, you have to scientifically map your pain level and trigger point to see how the pain changes and diminishes over time. Once you increase your awareness of these areas you can also better focus your mental healing imagery as well.

WHAT TO DO:

1. For this technique, use the same PFM description as outlined in the internal pelvic floor muscle myofascial release technique from earlier in this chapter.

2. Your objective is to find the painful trigger points in the PFMs and press them for 90 seconds until you eliminate the pain or decrease the pain by 50 percent.

3. You may have to press into the trigger points for several 90-second repetitions as one might not give you the relief right away. When you press on these painful spots avoid pressing too hard and stay below a pain level of 5 out of 10 (0= no pain, 10 = worst pain you ever had).

4. Many times the trigger points you find will refer pain to another part of your body. Remember that this is quite normal. Just continue to work hard to eliminate your trigger points as described above. When I find trigger points in my patients, I find areas that either have small bumps in them or feel raised or hard.

Internal Pelvic Floor Muscle Cross Friction Fiber Massage

GETTING STARTED:

Cross friction fiber massage requires a small motion, about half an inch to an inch of back and forth movement "across the fiber" of the pelvic floor muscles in a perpendicular motion. This technique is useful in places where you find pain, scar tissue, or bumps in the muscles. The amount of pressure should be moderate and really depends on your pain tolerance. This internal massage may cause some amount of discomfort, but it should never be too painful. I would avoid going over a level 5 pain (0 = no pain, 10 = worst pain ever) when performing this massage. Avoid massaging over the tendonous arch of the levator ani muscles. It will feel like a spaghetti noodle and almost always causes pain.

WHAT TO DO:

Diagram 9.3: Cross Friction Massage

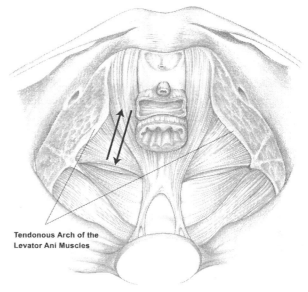

Tendonous Arch of the
Levator Ani Muscles

Arrows represent direction of massage with dilator or finger. Try to avoid the tendonous arch of the levator ani muscles, as it will almost always elicit pain.

1. Imagine again that the PFMs are a tube divided into 2 halves, a right half and a left half. The muscle fibers of the 2 halves generally run from superior to inferior, or top to bottom, and are parallel to each other. See diagram.

2. Massage across the PFM fiber in a perpendicular motion, which will be in an internal to external, or in to out motion across the muscle fiber, as in Diagram 9.3.

3. Insert your lubricated dilator or finger up to the third knuckle and start to search for painful muscle spots or spots that feel like there is a knot, scar or bumps in the muscle. Once you have identified a spot, use an internal to ex-

ternal massage stroke with either your finger or the tip of the dilator directly on the painful spot or across a bigger part of the muscle. For example, use an internal to external stroke at 3 o'clock in Layer 2 on the left side. Map your pain and track your progress.

4. Perform the cross friction massage for at least 3 to 5 minutes and then move to another location in the same side, if necessary. Cross friction massage helps to break down adhesions, spasms, and scar tissue, but it does take time.

5. I recommend that you wait at least 24 hours before doing the cross friction massage again just to see how you respond to this technique.

6. Keep track of your overall pain levels as this is your best gauge as to whether this method is good for you. You may have to try it a couple of times before determining if this method is the right one to incorporate into your healing program.

Internal Pelvic Floor Muscle Half–Moon Strumming Massage

GETTING STARTED:

Strumming is another great way to help release painful knots, spasms and trigger points in the PFMs. Strumming is similar to cross friction except that the motion is parallel, and goes along the muscle fiber. It is generally less painful than cross friction. Strumming and cross friction go hand-in-hand; you can mix and match the cross friction and strumming techniques based on your own internal palpation of your pelvic floor. Once you get used to your own muscles and locations of pain and spasm, you will begin to develop an intuition towards the best combination to alleviate your condition. Be your own detective, get to know your body, and listen to what your body is telling you. Tune into the messages that your body is sending, and you will be able to have better control.

Diagram 9.4: Half-Moon Strumming

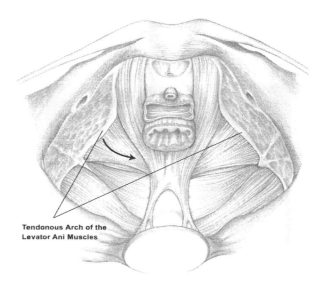

Tendonous Arch of the
Levator Ani Muscles

*Arrows represent direction of massage with dilator or finger. Try to avoid the tendonous
arch of the levator ani muscles, as it will almost always elicit pain.*

WHAT TO DO:

1. Strumming massage, as opposed to cross friction massage, is a type of
massage that is performed in the direction of the pelvic floor muscle fiber.
So this massage is from superior to inferior, or top to bottom.

2. First work the right half of the PFM and then work the left half, massaging
layer by layer from deepest Layer 3 to superficial Layer 1. For example, strum
from 3 to 4 o'clock in Layer 2 on the left side.

3. As with cross friction, always map your pain and techniques, so over time
you can get a good scientific sense of what is working.

4. Avoid masaging the arcus tendon of the levator ani muscle. It feels like
thick cooked spaghetti and will usually elicit pain.

Hand in hand with these internal techniques are the external massage and
release strategies discussed in the next chapter.

Chapter Ten

"If you want to reach a state of bliss, then go beyond your ego and the internal dialogue. Make a decision to relinquish the need to control, the need to be approved, and the need to judge. Those are the three things the ego is doing all the time. It's very important to be aware of them every time they come up."
—Deepak Chopra

Chapter 10

DECREASING PELVIC FLOOR MUSCLE PAIN WITH EXTERNAL HANDS-ON TECHNIQUES

Alongside your internal work, as discussed in Chapter 9, there are also some great ways to normalize PFM muscle and tissue function, flexibility, and range of motion that are done externally. I often recommend that my patients use these tools when they are having their periods and do not feel comfortable doing internal work. The external techniques are very effective in reducing pelvic pain symptoms. These techniques may help you locate and eliminate trigger points that could be referring pain to the PFMs and the hip/pelvic region. Also it helps to smooth out the muscle fibers and connective tissue that can easily contribute in subtle ways to your condition.

In Their Own Words - Healing My Pain Using Isa's Great Tools

"I came to Renew PT for pelvic pain syndrome called vulvodynia or vestibulitis. At Renew, I was given cold laser treatments and massages for specific muscles that were very tight or had trigger points in them. Isa also recorded my muscular tension with a machine that does biofeedback. In just over a month of twice weekly treatments, I am completely pain-free in huge part to Isa's treatment, but also from doing the homework she assigned me. I did these regularly even when I was traveling or could not make my appointments.

"Isa designed a program that included stretching, internal and external massages, and myofascial releases. What I like about Renew is that Isa approaches pelvic pain from multiple perspectives. It is not just muscular, neuropathic or stress related - she customizes a program to fit each individual person and then gives homework for empowerment. I highly recommend the excellent services and staff at Renew PT. I am here to say that I am pain-free because of their care."

General Guidelines

When doing these gentle massage techniques, watch out for the following:

1. You may experience muscle soreness 24 to 72 hours afterwards. This is normal.

2. These techniques can be very painful as you find spots that you may not have been aware of. Do not be alarmed, stay within a pain level of 3 to 5 rating. Back off, proceed slowly, and don't give up.

3. You may see some bruising on your skin after doing some of the rolling techniques. If this occurs, be gentler with the rolling, but do not become alarmed.

4. Your pelvic floor muscles may respond by tightening with some of these techniques. If this occurs, do your relax Kegel with diaphragmatic breathing and yoga Corpse Pose to calm everything down.

Table 10.1: External Techniques for Pelvic Muscle Release

NAME OF TECHNIQUE
1. Labia Stretch, Roll and Cross Friction Massage
2. Abdominal Rolling
3. Lower Back Massage
4. Sacral Rolling
5. Inner Thigh Massage and Trigger Point Release

Labia Stretch, Roll and Cross Friction Massage

GETTING STARTED:

This type of stretching and mobilization is great for women who are having pain with initial penetration or for women whose pelvic floor muscles are too tight and painful for intercourse. When performing these techniques, focus on increasing the flexibility and suppleness of the labial tissue. These techniques are also great to use when you have your period and do not want to do internal work.

WHAT TO DO:

Labia Stretch

Anchor your finger on the top of the right labia majora near the clitoris. With the thumb of the opposite hand, place it at the bottom of the same labia and stretch downward, hold for 30 seconds to 1 minute, repeating 2 to 3 times and then switch to the other labia.

Diagram 10.1: Labia Stretch

Labia Roll

Pinch the right labia majora between the thumb and the forefinger. Roll the tissue gently between the fingers until you reach the bottom. Repeat 2 to 3 times and then switch sides.

Diagram 10.2 : Labia Cross Friction Massage

Labia Cross Friction Massage

Place your index or forefinger on the top of your right labia majora. Gently massage the tissue across the labia from side to side until you reach the bottom. Repeat 2 to 3 times and then switch sides.

Abdominal Rolling

GETTING STARTED:

The PFMs are connected to the fascia of the abdominal muscles. When the PFMs are painful, in spasms, and lack mobility, the abdominal muscle can sometimes respond by becoming tight, painful and developing trigger points in them also. I find that when abdominal massage and rolling are incorporated into the treatment sessions, my patients are better able to tolerate the intra-vaginal stretches and massage more easily. Many of my patients tell me that after the abdominal massage they can insert their dilator or finger with more ease and less pain. The abdominal muscles may also have trigger points in them, and you will discover yours as you massage the abdominals.

If you came across a very painful trigger point (and sometimes these painful spots can refer pain elsewhere in the pelvis, hold the spot for 90 seconds until the pain subsides. Repeat the 90-second holds until you have either eliminated the trigger point or reduced the pain by 50 percent. Remember it's important to determine your pain level at the start of any treatment so that you can track your progress. To facilitate abdominal rolling, place a heating pad or hot water bottle on your tummy for 10 minutes before you start your rolling.

Precaution for Abdominal Rolling

Your physician will provide the guidelines, but generally you must wait until 6 weeks after your abdominal surgery or C-section before starting these techniques. This is when the abdominal scar is almost fully healed. Your doctor may give you permission to start earlier, but you must be cleared by your doctor before starting abdominal rolling/massage before 6 weeks.

WHAT TO DO:

1. Get a nice aromatherapy oil with a scent that helps you to relax as you work with your abdominal rolling

2. Cup your abdominal muscles by placing index fingers near each other so they are gently touching and place your thumbs superior to the other fingers as in the photo on page 179. Stay superficial on your abdominal muscle and avoid grabbing the muscles too deeply.

3. Gently glide your fingers towards your thumbs repeating 10 to 20 times and change your hand placement. For simplicity's sake, I have divided the abdominal muscles into an upper part and lower part. Roll the lower part first, focusing on upward motions. Make sure to cover all the lower abdominal muscles and then switch to rolling the upper abdominal muscles in a downward motion.

4. Remember to pay attention to the trigger points and handle or treat them as previously described in this chapter.

5. End your abdominal rolling by gently massaging your entire abdominal region with clockwise circles.

6. Try to roll your abdominals 5 to 15 minutes on a daily basis and perform at least 20 clockwise circles to end your massage.

Lower Back Massage

GETTING STARTED:

Many of the women I treat with pelvic pain also suffer from lower back pain. These two conditions go hand in hand. Massaging the lower back is important to help release tension and trigger points in this region.

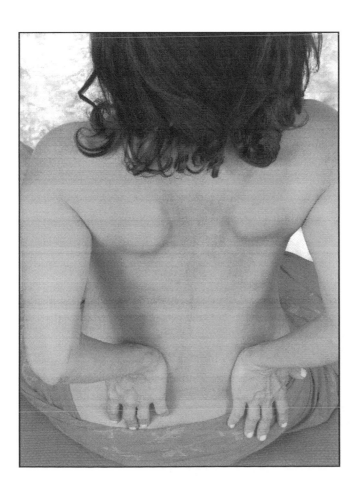

WHAT TO DO:

1. Learn to massage yourself in different positions and use firm pressure avoiding excessive pain.

2. Massage down the lower back muscles using long downward strokes. You can use your knuckles or hands. Make sure to cover the entire lower back area.

3. Using your right hand, massage your right lower back muscles for 5 to 10 minutes. Then switch sides massaging your left lower back muscles with your left hand.

4. For painful trigger points found in any of the back muscles, apply sustained pressure over the painful area for 90 seconds. Repeat as necessary until the pain has decreased by at least 50 percent or the pain is totally eliminated.

5. A great addition to the low back rolling is to massage your low back outward from the spine along the line of your hip bone using your knuckles. This can be very painful at first, but continue to do this massage until the pain has diminished by 50 percent.

Sacral Rolling

GETTING STARTED:

The sacrum houses many of the nerve roots that innervate the abdominal organs, PFMs and hip muscles. It is of critical importance to keep the tissues in this area free and supple. One of the great tools that I give my patients is sacral rolling.

WHAT TO DO:

1. Basically cup the skin in your sacral area and roll it in the same man-

ner that you would roll your abdominals. See the photo for hand placement.

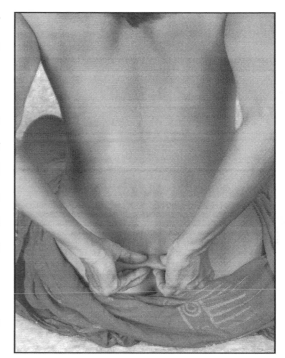

2. Roll the sacrum upwards for 2 to 5 minutes on a daily basis. In the beginning, sacral rolling might be painful to do but over time as you roll the sacrum it will become less painful to do.

3. The goal is to be pain-free when doing the sacral rolling.

Inner Thigh Massage, Rolling and Trigger Point Release

GETTING STARTED:

The inner thigh muscles require special attention because of their close proximity to the pelvis and PFMs. The inner thigh muscles can develop spasms, trigger points and adhesions in them as a response to what is happening internally in the PFMs. These tissue abnormalities can make sitting, walking and positional changes painful. To restore proper function, muscle length, and flexibility to the inner thigh muscles, use the three techniques described below.

Long Deep Inner Thigh Strokes

WHAT TO DO:

1. Massage the inner thigh muscles from the knee to the upper groin, using long deep strokes for 5 to 10 minutes.

2. If performing the massage without oil is too painful, you can use a small drop of oil or massage cream to make the gliding less painful.

Inner Thigh Skin Rolling
WHAT TO DO:

1. Roll your inner thigh muscles from the knee to the groin using the rolling techniques described under abdominal rolling.

2. Roll the inner thigh for 10 to 5 minutes or as tolerated.

Inner Thigh Trigger Point Release
WHAT TO DO:

1. The inner thigh muscles can develop trigger points in them as a response to pelvic pain. Search for these trigger points by running your hands slowly along your inner thigh muscles. A trigger point will feel like a hard, small ball and will produce pain when touched.

2. Once you find them, press into the trigger points for 90 seconds until the pain has diminished or gone away. You may have to do several cycles of 90 seconds to accomplish this.

The internal and external techniques outlined in the last 2 chapters are some of the most important keys to your overall success. If your pain has a post-surgical scar component as well, add the scar-care mobilizations in the next chapter to ensure your success.

Chapter Eleven

"There are as many nights as days, and the one is just as long as the other in the year's course. Even a happy life cannot be without a measure of darkness, and the word 'happy' would lose its meaning if it were not balanced by sadness."
- Carl Jung

Chapter 11

SCAR-CARE TECHNIQUES: INTRODUCTION

As outlined in Chapter 2, post-surgical scar adhesions occur in women after most pelvic, abdominal, and C-section surgeries. The fibrous bands that form during the healing process post surgery often cause tissues to grow together that normally would not be connected. In my experience, the longer a woman waits to seek therapy for her scars, the denser and tougher the scar adhesions become. I have seen women develop pelvic and sexual pain as a result of abdominal surgeries for fibroids, hysterectomy, C-sections, and endometriosis, even though there were no incisions made in the pelvic floor muscles.

New mothers are one group of women that tend to be overlooked and often not even classified as post-operative. I treat many post-partum women at my healing center who have had significant perineal tears or episiotomies during their labor, who then come to me complaining about sexual pain. Their common complaint is that they are not "the same down there." Sometimes they tell me their husbands no longer fit inside them. Many of these new mothers have significant sexual pain, pain with walking, and/or pain with sitting. Recent research has shown that one out of three women have sexual pain a year after giving birth. Many of these young mothers also complain that they have trouble with breastfeeding and taking care of their young infants because of their abdominal or perineal scar pain. Many patients tell me that they have heard there is nothing you can do to alleviate these conditions, and are often told things like "Welcome to motherhood."

Another group of women often overlooked are those who have undergone C-sections. The statistics show that over 31 percent of births in the US are done by C-section. Make no mistake: a C-section is a major surgery. Adhesions, pelvic and sexual pain are often a direct result of scars that have become bound down. I often see C-section patients who have developed vulvodynia and pelvic floor muscle dysfunction as a result of the surgery.

Women who have experienced any of the above surgical procedures will benefit from stretching and mobilizing their scars to prevent scar adhesions. Many women who come to me have no idea how to care for their scars. In particular women who undergo C-sections or other abdominal surgeries are often not given advice on how to care for their scars when they leave the hospital. Some may even feel ashamed of their C-section scars because they feel a sense of failure over not having the vaginal birth.

Many women are afraid to touch their scars and experience problems because their scars are bound down, inflexible and have multiple dense adhesions. Furthermore, post-surgical patients often complain to me about upper and lower back and neck pain. I find many of these spinal pains are related to postural problems because their scars are pulling their bodies inward and forward, causing trigger points and spasms in the scars and muscles. Some of my patients also complain about not being able to wear certain clothes. Many tell me they feel changes in the weather in their scars. The critical thing to remember is that post-surgical scars must be dealt with and that scar pain and adhesions must be resolved as part of the solution in the journey to regain normal functioning and pain-free intimacy.

Before undertaking any of the scar therapy techniques in this chapter, it is critical to look at Table 11.1 for warning signs and precautions. Make sure to check with your doctor or birth caregiver to get their approval before starting any of the scar techniques and massages. When in doubt about a technique, seek help from a healthcare professional such as a physical therapist who specializes in pelvic floor and scar conditions to make sure you get on the right track.

In Their Own Words - Post-Partum Scar Pain; 4th Degree Tear

"I came to Renew Physical Therapy to see Isa because I had post-partum scar pain from 3 surgical repairs. During the birth of my child I experienced a 4th-degree tear to my perineum and rectum. I felt very weak and wanted to be stronger. My doctor said I was perfectly healed, but I was still in so much pain. He said this was normal and to be expected, so I believed him. For 2 months I tried to ignore the pain, so when I came to see Isa and she asked me if I had any pain, I said no. I really wasn't connected to my pelvic muscles, so I thought I had no pain.

"Isa taught me how to keep track of my pain in a journal even though I told her I just came to retrain and strengthen my muscles. With my journal on hand at my next appointment, I realized that not only did I have pain, but I had extreme pain all day, in every situation! I had pain with sitting and had pain with sex. Wearing my thong underwear also hurt.

"I have been seeing Isa for about 2 months now and she worked with me to strengthen, stretch and mobilize my scar tissue. We worked both on the vaginal and rectal tissues. She used laser therapy as well which was amazing, I literally walked out of the healing center with no pain the first time she did it. Each time after that, I just got better and better. Now, after 2 months, I feel stronger than even before I had my son. I am almost pain-free. I am able to wear clothes without any difficulty, including my tight jeans and thong underwear without pain.

"I highly recommend physical therapy at Renew PT for women who have had a baby – whether they were injured or not or had a C-section or not - to get better and stronger. A lot of times, we are unaware of what is happening in our bodies until someone focuses on it. I am really thankful for Renew Physical Therapy."

Table11.1: Precautions for Abdominal and Perineal Scar Therapy

TYPE OF PRECAUTION
1. If you have recently had surgery, get clearance from your medical doctor before starting the vaginal and abdominal techniques in this chapter.
2. If you have recently given birth and have an episiotomy, perineal tear and/or perineal repair, get clearance from your midwife or medical doctor before starting the vaginal techniques, dilator stretches or abdominal scar therapy outlined in this chapter.
3. Proceed with caution if you have undergone abdominal surgeries. Check with your doctor to make sure that the scar therapy and massage techniques in this book are appropriate for your recovery.
4. Avoid the techniques in this chapter if you have a vaginal infection, abdominal scar infection or bleeding from the vagina or abdominal scar.
5. Avoid abdominal scar massage if your scar is oozing fluids. Inform your caregiver about any changes to your scars.
6. If you have recently given birth, wait 6 weeks before massaging perineal and c section scars and get medical clearance first from your midwife or doctor.
7. Report any increase in scar pain to your caregiver, and have your doctor check to make sure the scar is healing well.
8. Immediately report to your caregiver any foul-smelling odor coming from your vagina, abdominal or perineal scar as this could be a sign of infection.
9. Always start gently and superficially with all massage techniques listed in this chapter. Discontinue if the scar becomes painful.
10. I recommend getting expert advice from a women's health physiotherapist to make sure you are performing the techniques correctly.
11. You can massage the scar as soon as the Steri-Strips fall off. Only masage the areas of the scar that are healed completely. Don't massage parts of the scar that are open or oozing.
12. If you are unsure about the techniques, wait until your 6 week checkup before starting or continuing the techniques in this chapter.

Scar Massage Therapy Basics

Massaging scars, whether in the perineum or abdominal area, helps to restore proper function to the muscles, increase blood circulation to the muscles, promote better scar healing, and prevent adhesions from becoming too tough or dense. If you have a C-section scar, a myomectomy or other abdominal scar, it is usually alright to start gently massaging an abdominal scar as soon as the Steri-Strips have fallen off, and you have approval from your doctor.

If you have any doubts about massaging the scar, consult your physician and/or caregiver about when to start. Different surgical procedures heal at different rates. Many doctors have their own protocols as to when the scar therapy can start. You will always derive benefits with proper massage of your scar, but YOU MUST GET CLEARANCE from your doctor BEFORE STARTING any scar massage techniques to avoid altering the surgical procedure and possibly damaging the tissues. For these scar massage techniques, you can use massage cream once your doctor or caregiver gives the green light. You can also use scar oils or ointments such as Mederma, scar guard, vitamin E, or even plain olive oil to do your massages.

Table 11.2: Scar Therapy Techniques for the Relief of Pain and Adhesions

TECHNIQUE
1. Scar Trigger Point Release
2. Abdominal Scar Massage Long Strokes
3. Deeper Scar Massage: Clockwise Circles
4. Abdominal Scar Lift
5. Abdominal Scar Rolling
6. Scar Stretching Techniques – Longitudinal
7. Scar Down and X-Pattern
8. Perineal/Vaginal Massage Therapy

Scar Trigger Point Release

WHAT TO DO:

1. Check the length of the scar and press gently along it looking for spots that elicit pain when touched or that refer pain to another location.

2. Once a painful spot is found, gently press into it, holding the spot without releasing the pressure for 60 to 90 seconds. Repeat 2 to 3 times until the pain has diminished. Repeat the point pressure therapy several times until the scar pain is reduced by 50 percent. You can apply pressure on the same spot for several 60 to 90 second repetitions until the pain has subsided.

3. Avoid pressing into the scar too aggressively. Grade your pressure and press into the scar to a tolerable pain level. Pressing into the scar too hard will cause the PFM to tighten in response to the scar pain.

4. While you are doing your scar point pressure therapy, pay attention to your pelvic floor muscles and make sure to keep them relaxed. Also, to deal with the pain, it helps to breath diaphragmatically, with long deep breaths, in through the nose and out through the mouth.

Abdominal Scar Massage Long Strokes

WHAT TO DO:

1. To restore flexibility to an abdominal or C-section scar, massage it using long strokes along the length of the scar.

2. Perform 20 long strokes from left to right across the scar superficially at first and then as the pain decreases, go deeper until you are at the layer of the adhesions.

3. Repeat with 20 long strokes from right to left.

Deeper Scar Massage: Clockwise Circles

WHAT TO DO:

1. Perform small clockwise circles along the scar from right to left, using different graded pressure as tolerated. Start superficially and then go deeper as you are able. Repeat with small circles from left to right.

Abdominal Scar Lift

WHAT TO DO:

1. Divide the scar into small areas. Starting on one side, pick up the scar between your index finger and thumb. Try to pick up some of the underlying scar tissue, not just the outer layer of skin.

2. Once you pick up the scar and some of the underlying tissue, hold it for 30 seconds before moving across to the next section. If needed, you can hold the upward lift longer and wait for the scar to release. The release will feel like the scar is lengthening naturally.

Abdominal Scar Rolling

WHAT TO DO:

1. Pick up the scar along its length and roll it between your thumb and index finger. This might be very difficult to do if the scar is bound down or inflexible.

2. If the scar does not lift up, do not be alarmed. Your goal is to break up the adhesions and to be able to lift up the skin of the scar.

Scar Stretching Techniques – Longitudinal, Scar Down, X-Pattern

GETTING STARTED:

Just like other muscles in the body, scars can benefit immensely from being stretched. There are three main types of stretching I recommend to my patients that provide the most relief, but do not attempt to do scar stretching unless you get clearance from your doctor or caregiver.

Longitudinal Scar Stretch

WHAT TO DO:

1. Hold down the left side of the scar and with your left hand, stretch the scar by pulling it to the right with your right hand until you feel resistance.

2. Hold the stretch for 30 to 60 seconds.

3. Repeat 2 to 5 times, then switch sides.

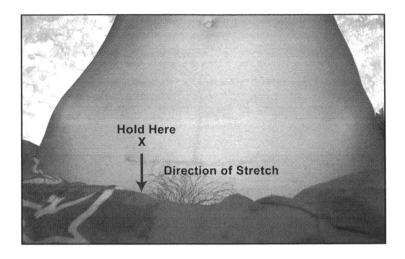

Scar Down Stretch

WHAT TO DO:

1. Place your right index finger on top of the scar about a half inch away from the scar and place your left index finger below the scar in a straight line.

2. Hold the right index finger in place and gently use the left finger to stretch the scar in a linear pattern as if you were trying to pull the scar apart.

3. Continue this stretching along the scar from right to left and from left to right, as shown in the photo.

X Pattern Scar Stretch

WHAT TO DO:

1. Place your right index finger on top of the scar about a half inch away from the scar and place your left index finger diagonally below the scar.

2. Pull the fingers away from each other, thereby stretching the scar. Hold this stretch for 5 seconds, then switch hands. Place your left index finger above the scar and your right index finger below the scar and pull the fingers away from each other, holding for another 5 seconds.

3. This type of stretching creates an X pattern. Perform this X pattern along the scar first, from right to left and then left to right.

Perineal/Vaginal Massage Therapy

Many of the women I treat have pelvic pain resulting from an episiotomy or a perineal tear during the delivery of their child. When they come to see me they are in a state of depression and anxiety. Not only do they have a newborn at home that requires their undivided attention but now they also have to endure pain while sitting, standing, and in many cases simply changing positions. Other women who can benefit from this type of stretching include those who have undergone biopsies, vestibulodectomy, or reconstructive surgeries.

For the perineal/vaginal scar therapy, it is helpful to use a mirror to look and examine the scar before stretching and mobilizing the scar. The following massage routines are great techniques that can be used to alleviate painful scars in the perineum. These methods can also be used to help mobilize and make the pelvic floor muscles more supple, flexible and pain-free. These techniques work great for women who are on a healing journey to pain-free intimacy, and can be used even if you don't have a scar.

Perineal Scar Rolling

WHAT TO DO:

1. Place the scar between the fingers tips. You might have to place one finger inside the vagina and one finger outside the vagina, gently gripping the scar between the fingertips in order to roll it.

2. Roll the scar between your fingers for 2 to 3 minutes or as tolerated until the scar feels loose, less painful and more pliable. Perineal scar rolling is a great method to get the scar more flexible and mobile.

Perineal Body Massage

Base Image: Netter Images

WHAT TO DO:

1. Use the trigger point release techniques as outlined earlier in Part III, but this time on the perineal body.

2. Once you locate a painful area or trigger point, push on that spot for 90 seconds.

3. For best results, try pressing into the perineal body at different angles and locations in the perineum. Hold each different direction for 20 to 30 seconds.

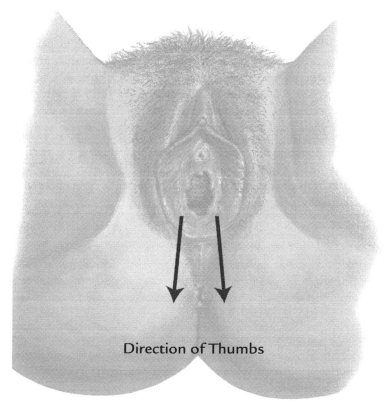

Direction of Thumbs

Base Image: Netter Images

Traditional Perineal Thumb Massage

GETTING STARTED:

This massage method works great for perineal scars, for pelvic pain sufferers with vaginismus, and also as a preparation for labor and delivery. Pregnant women can start this massage on the 34th week of pregnancy for 3 to 5 minutes. Make sure to check with your obstetrician, gynecologist or midwife before starting the perineal massage. I often teach my pregnant patients' partners to do this massage to help them prepare for labor.

WHAT TO DO:

1. Lubricate your thumbs, insert them into the vagina up to the first knuckle, and press straight downward towards the rectum for 3 to 5 minutes.

2. After 3 to 5 minutes, press down to the right for several seconds and then to the left for several seconds.

3. Another technique is to do half-moon strokes with your thumbs. Place your right thumb up to the first knuckle in the inside of your left pelvic floor muscles. Start from top to bottom performing half-moon strokes from the top to bottom for about one minute, then change sides and perform the half-moon strokes on the other side.

So far we have covered a lot of ground and I've presented many techniques that you can incorporate as you work hard to reduce your symptoms. Remember, as I mentioned in Part I, you have to get on a road that will transform every aspect of your life. This includes having at your disposal a set of tools and information that you will use in times when you are not stretching, exercising, massaging, and mobilizing your pelvic floor muscles.

The tools and techniques that you will read about next in Part IV are great tips and strategies that can bring soothing comfort and relief for irritated skin, painful flare-ups and muscle spasms. You also need to pull together an all-encompassing mind-body approach with daily meditations, visualizations, and affirmations to break the cycle of self-blame, shame, and hopelessness that often accompanies conditions involving the PFMs.

Again, as in Part III, there is no set order or series outlined in this next section as in the stretching and strengthening series. I have merely put together a pelvic pain relief toolbox for you filled with my most tried and true techniques and remedies that my patients tell me give them the most relief and motivation to continue on their journeys to pain-free living.

Part 4
Pelvic Pain Relief Toolbox

"When it is dark enough, you can see the stars."
— *Ralph Waldo Emerson*

Chapter 12

BASIC TOOLS FOR BETTER VULVAR SKIN CARE

When my patients come to see me at my center I always ask them, "When was the last time you examined your vagina?" Almost always, the answer varies from never to several months. I think it's safe to say that most women are not taught vulva-vaginal health, self-care and self-examination. As a child, the only vulvar care/hygiene I learned was to wipe from front to back. Proper vulvar care, hygiene, and self-examination are great ways to understand your unique anatomy, understand what is normal for you, and are essential in monitoring your vulvar health. The importance of performing monthly vulvar self-exam cannot be stressed enough, which is why I dedicated a whole section of this book in Part I to vaginal self-examination. I've seen several different physicians in the past several years and not once was I instructed on how to do this exam.

Remember, as we discussed in Part I, you will do your self-exam at least once a month and take note of any changes. Track issues like skin irritation, changes in coloration, discharge, pain levels and locations, and any other relevant information that will help you get a better understanding of your pelvic floor. If you are experiencing burning, itching, or irritation, use some of the great remedies listed in this chapter to get some relief. If your condition persists, make sure you work with a doctor who can help make some specific recommendations as well. The techniques I am presenting in this chapter are by no means a substitute for proper medical care.

Basic Vulvar Skin Hygiene

Irritation and burning of the vulva and vagina are common among women suffering from pelvic pain conditions. There are many things you can do to minimize these feelings in your vulva. The following is a list of recommendations that have worked for my patients. Remember, these are only recommendations and you must find the ones that are appropriate for you and your condition. If you have any doubt, please show the list to your caregiver to make sure that you are practicing the ones that will work best for you.

Recommendations for Better Vulvar Care

1. Although it may seem obvious, always wipe from front to back after urination and bowel movement to avoid infections.

2. Keep the vulva area dry. Pat dry the vulva; do not vigorously rub it with towels or toilet paper. If the vulva is irritated, use a blow drier set on cool or let it air dry.

3. Sleep in the nude at night. My patients find sleeping in the nude helps reduce their irritation.

4. Avoid irritants such as perfumed soaps, bubble bath, feminine hygiene products and colored toilet paper on the vulva. If you must use soap, try something gentle and fragrance-free or try calendula soap. Also avoid getting shampoo on the vulva.

5. Use unscented white and chlorine-free toilet paper, and whenever possible, use organic toilet paper.

6. Use menstrual pads and tampons that are perfume-free and 100 percent cotton. Make sure to use the appropriate tampon size for menstrual flow.

During light days, use tampons with lighter absorbency, and during heavy days use super absorbency. Again whenever possible, use organic products and avoid deodorized sanitary pads and tampons.

7. Avoid pushing with urination and defecation. Avoid constipation by drinking enough water for proper hydration and taking in enough fiber. Staying properly hydrated helps keep the urine diluted and makes it less likely to irritate the vulva and the bladder.

8. After urinating, rinse the vulva with cool to lukewarm water. A perineal bottle (spray bottle) works great. Alternatively, you can invest in a bidet for your home. Using a perineal bottle is especially great after childbirth.

9. Avoid douches unless prescribed by your caregiver. Douches can upset the natural balance of organisms in the vagina.

10. Avoid chlorinated water and avoid swimming in pools. I've had patients flare-up terribly after being in chlorinated pools.

11. Perform vaginal steams as described later in Part IV once a week and the day after your menstrual cycle ends.

Helpful Tips for Relieving Vulvar Pain

1. A&D™ Ointment for babies works great on irritated vulvar skin. Apply a small amount of A&D™ Ointment to the vulva as needed to protect the skin. A&D™ also works great for women who experience increased friction in the vulvar area with walking.

2. Calendula cream applied to the vulvar area will help soothe irritated skin. Use on another body part first to make sure you are not allergic to it.

Calendula is derived from a flower and is used to soothe skin inflammation. You can also use a calendula wash and soap, which is described later in this chapter.

3. Too many times my patients use over-the-counter anti-yeast treatments only to make the burning and irritation worst. Do not use over-the-counter creams, ointments and anti-yeast medications without consulting your caregiver first. Prescription medications like Diflucan™ can also get rid of yeast infections without irritation to the vulva-vaginal area.

4. To soothe vulvar burning, some women find relief by using witch hazel pads (TUCKS Pads) to areas of discomfort. These pads are also a lifesaver after giving birth.

5. Taking lukewarm to warm baths helps with vulvar itching and burning. Fill the bath tub with a few inches of lukewarm to warm water and add colloidal oatmeal such as Aveeno™ to help reduce itching. If the Aveeno™ doesn't help, then try adding 4 to 5 tablespoons of baking soda to the bath to soothe vulvar itching and irritation.

6. Use sitz baths to relieve burning and irritation. A sitz bath is a bath in which the hips and buttock are submerged. Usually a small basin is used and placed on top of the toilet. After childbirth, using a sitz bath with Epsom salt can really help reduce pain and prevent infections. You can also steep calendula flowers and add the calendula water to your bath as well.

7. Apply a cool compress for 10 to 15 minutes to the vulva to help decrease pain and irritation. This technique is great if you have had a recent flare-up or severe vulvar pain.

Common Treatments for Perineal Vulvar Health

The perineum is an extremely sensitive area of the vulvar region that often undergoes trauma, especially during childbirth, when women may experience perineal tearing and episiotomies. Sometimes these wounds do not heal properly or do not heal at all, and continue to open up with intercourse, defecation and exercise. For persistent perineal wounds that do not seem to heal properly, work with your doctor or caregiver to find the right combination of medicines and vitamins that will complement your perineal stretching and scar mobilizations that I've outlined in Part III. The following is a list of remedies that my patients have tried with positive results, but make sure to work with your doctor to be certain of the combination that is right for your specific needs.

Vitamins to Improve Skin Conditions of the Perineum

To be taken internally and under the supervision a healthcare professional

1. Vitamin C
2. Vitamin A
3. Vitamin D
4. Vitamin E

Alternative Massage Oils and Creams for the Perineum

1. Vitamin E oil – Organic if possible
2. Rose oil
3. Wild yam cream
4. Sesame Oil
5. Yoni cream
6. Calendula cream

Doctor-Prescribed Topical Creams and Medicines for the Perineum

1. Estrogen/Lidocaine combo

2. Testosterone cream

3. Estrogen/testosterone combo

4. Lidocaine

5. Steroidal cream

6. Elavil™

7. Muscle relaxers

8. Valium™

9. Estrogen E-ring for dryness of vagina, called atrophic vaginitis

10. Vagifem

11. Botox - internal injection

Vulvar Care and Clothing

1. Avoid wearing pantyhose. Use thigh or knee-high hose instead. If you must wear pantyhose, cut the crotch out.

2. Double rinse any clothes that come in contact with the vulva. Wash clothes with mild fragrance-free detergents such as Dreft™ or Seventh Generation™. Avoid fabric softeners and dryer sheets on all clothing that comes in contact with the vulvar area. Whenever possible use organic, fragrance-free detergents.

3. Remove wet clothing immediately, especially after swimming and wash the vulvar area with water as soon as possible to avoid burning and inflammation that many times comes with swimming in a chlorinated pool.

4. Avoid wearing very tight jeans and pants and clothes made from synthetic fabrics that capture sweat and increase irritation. Also avoid low-rider jeans that can put pressure on the bladder area. Instead choose a pair of jeans that are loose and baggy in the crotch area of the pants and are loose around the waist.

5. Try wearing 100 percent cotton underwear. Many of my patients find that thongs increase vulvar irritation and many times also irritate the anal area.

Managing Vulvar Pain after Sexual Intercourse

1. Use water-soluble lubricants for sexual intercourse. When possible, use only organic products.

2. Urinate after sex.

3. Rinse the vulva with cool water after sex.

4. Apply a cold compress to the vulva immediately after sex to reduce irritation. Apply compress for at least 15 to 20 minutes for better results. Repeat every hour as necessary.

5. Lidocaine, commonly prescribed by doctors, helps reduce pain during sex. Lidocaine can sometimes burn for 3 to 5 minutes after application.

6. Focus on outercourse or tantric sex instead of intercourse when you are in pain. Experiment with lap dancing, oral sex, massage, mutual masturbation. Old-fashioned kissing can go a long way when you cannot have sexual intercourse.

7. If you are having intercourse, make sure you are both fully aroused and well-lubricated to reduce the actual penetration time and pain.

8. Make sure to do reverse Kegels before sexual penetration to reduce pain. Too many times my patients contract their muscles out of fear or habit right before intercourse, which increases their pain.

9. Experiment with different sexual positions to see which ones are the least painful.

10. Perform manual stretching with your finger or dilator before sex as highlighted in Part III of this book. This will allow the muscles to be more supple and relaxed.

Exercise and Vulvar Care

1. Avoid exercise that puts direct pressure on the vulva, such as biking and horseback riding. If you must bike, use padded pants and a padded seat or a bike seat designed to alleviate pressure on the pelvis such as the BiSaddle™, which has two mini seats built into one. Also try to limit the length of time you spend biking in general.

2. Low-impact exercises such as walking are great because they don't create a lot of friction in the vaginal area. For some, walking is not enough for them to really get their hearts pumping. High-impact exercises are acceptable as long as they don't increase your vulvar or vaginal discomfort. The best advice is to find cardiovascular exercises that don't increase gluteal, hip, or low-back muscle spasms, and especially vaginal pain. Cardiovascular exercise is important to do on a daily basis as it helps decrease stress, elevate natural endorphin levels (natural pain killers), and keep the heart and mind healthy. However, you have to find a balance so you don't worsen any painful symptoms.

3. Avoid exercising in highly synthetic materials that do not breathe and instead capture sweat. These types of materials increase vulvar irritation. Use cotton materials. Wear loose-fitting clothes and change your underwear immediately after exercise.

4. Perform the techniques in this book on a daily basis, especially the PFM stretching which will help reduce your pelvic pain.

5. Use a cool pack or ice pack on the vulva after exercising if pain increases. Wrap the cool pack up with 1 to 3 towels so that you don't cause damage to this very gentle skin. Cool packs and ice packs can be left on for 15 to 20 minutes.

6. Avoid classes like spinning and kickboxing which can throw out your hip and sacral alignment and put excessive pressure on the perineum. Practice your reverse Kegels as instructed in Part II so you can maintain your focus on your pelvic floor as you do your exercises.

Vaginal Steams for Vulvar/Vaginal Health and to Decrease Pain

Many of my patients swear by their vaginal steams and get great results with them. They experience less pain with sitting, have easier penetration, and are able to perform their vaginal stretches and insert dilators with more ease. I recommend doing vaginal steams on a weekly basis and even more often during painful flare-ups. Vaginal steams heat the pelvic floor muscles and help reduce tightness and muscle spasms. Vaginal steams should be avoided during your menstrual period or during pregnancy.

I recently treated a woman with a 10-year history of vaginismus. She had graduated to the largest dilator after several months of therapy, but was still experiencing pain and difficulty with its insertion. I recommended that she do a vaginal steam right before her dilator work. The following week she came to my office and was joyous. After her vaginal steam, she was able to insert the largest dilator without any problems. She said, "The dilator went right in, and I also had so much less pain with insertion."

Vaginal steams were taught to me by Dr. Rosita Arvigo, naturopathic doctor, renowned herbalist and Mayan healer. She has brought Maya Abdominal Massage to the United States and runs a great advanced certification program in Belize which I've completed. I find that many of the techniques of the Maya massage are essential for pelvic pain sufferers. The Arvigo Maya Abdominal Massage™ helps to realign the pelvic organs and decreases pelvic congestion by bringing healing energy and blood flow to the pelvic organs and pelvic floor muscles. With vaginal steams, you can mix and match the herbs and flowers you use depending on your condition. Consult a local herbalist before attempting to do a steam with herbs. Start your search on the web by checking out *www.ArvigoMassage.com*. You can also just start out with plain steamed water for the vaginal steams and still get results.

Vaginal Steam Instructions

1. Boil a gallon of water for 10 minutes and then let it steep with the herbs for 5 minutes with the lid on the pot.

2. Place water under a chair with open slits, or better yet place the bowl with the herbs into the toilet. Don't pour the steam solution into the toilet. Instead, put the whole pot into the toilet. Be careful as it might be too hot when you sit. If it feels too hot, you can also buy a raised toilet seat to avoid burns from the steam to the vulvar area/PFM.

3. Sit on the toilet and let the steam penetrate the PFMs via the vagina. If the steam is too hot, stand up and wait for it to cool down before sitting down again.

4. Wrap yourself in a blanket, put on socks, and make sure to avoid drafts while you are doing the steam. Sit down until all the steam has evaporated, about 15 to 20 minutes.

5. While sitting on the toilet, perform a reverse Kegel so that the pelvic muscles are evenly heated and relaxed. The steam introduces heat into the pelvic muscles, helping them to relax and reduce spasms of the pelvic floor muscles.

6. Add to your vaginal steam water a mixture of dry flower and herbs. Dr. Arvigo has made a wonderful healing remedy for vaginal steams, using herbs and flowers like basil, oregano, calendula flowers and lavender.

7. After the vaginal steam, massage the vaginal muscles. This is also a great time to insert your dilator and rest in bed under warm sheets. Do your best after a steam to keep your body at a constant warm temperature for 24 hours, avoiding sudden drafts that might give you a chill.

8. Work with a local herbalist to see which flower/herb mixture might be the best for the specifics of your condition. See the following table for herbs and their uses. You will need one quart of the herbs if you are using fresh herbs and one cup if using dry herbs.

Table 12.1: Herbs That Can Be Used in Your Vaginal Steams

Note: This list is for educational purposes only. You must consult your physician or herbalist before using any of these herbs in a vaginal steam. These herbs should not be taken by pregnant and lactating women unless prescribed by your caregiver. The information in this table comes from www.mountainroseherbs.com.

NAME OF HERB	USES
Calendula	Helps to reduce pain naturally. Its antibacterial, antinflammatory, antfungal, and immunostimulant properties help treat slow-healing cuts. It soothes irritated, burning skin and also helps to stimulate collagen synthesis.
Basil	Helps restore immune function deficiency caused by stress. It also has antibacterial properties and helps other herbs penetrate the skin.

NAME OF HERB	USES
Motherwort	Helps with menstrual tension by acting as a uterine tonic. This herb has antibacterial, antifungal, antispasmodic, anti-viral, and antiseptic properties.
Oregano	This herb has antispasmodic, antiviral, and antiseptic properties.
Rosemary	Has antioxidant, antiseptic, and antispasmodic properties. Helps to stop yeast from growing and helps to remove yeast cells from the urinary tract. Stimulates menstrual flow. Avoid this herb if your flow is already heavy.
St. John's Wort	Helps relieve pain. Should not be used together with Monoamine Oxidase Inhibitors (MAOIs) or Protease Inhibitors(PIs). Also helps to slow down frequent urination, and can treat throbbing pain of any origin.
Chamomile	Helps stop spasms in the smooth muscles and contains antiinflammatory, antibacterial, antiviral, and antiparasitic properties.
Red Clover	Helps reduce pain associated with menstrual periods. Helps promote healing of skin wounds and reduces the effects of PMS and menopause. Avoid this herb if you are taking a blood thinner.
Marshmallow Root	Relieves irritation by coating inflamed surfaces; relieves vulva, perineal, and vestibular inflammation.

Daily Warm Baths to Relieve Muscle Spasms

One of the key recommendations that I make to my patients suffering from vaginal and PFM pain is warm baths. Not only do warm baths help reduce muscle spasms, but they also help reduce stress and anxiety. I recommend two baths a day, one before work and another at the end of the day right before going to bed. Make sure the bath water is not too hot and fill the tub so that your abdominals are entirely covered by the water. You may have to make the water less hot if you are having vulvar skin irritation. If tolerated, try adding Epsom salt or sea salt to the bath water. These salts help relax the muscles and thereby help to lower your pain naturally.

Calendula Wash

WHAT TO DO:

1. Boil a handful of calendula in 2 cups of water.

2. Let the mixture stand for 30 minutes or until the water turns amber.

3. Wait until the solution is room temperature, then add to your tub or sitz bath. If possible, sit for 30 minutes in your calendula bath.

4. During the immediate post-partum period, put the calendula wash into a perineal spritz bottle and use it to rinse the vulva after urination.

Ice/Heat Packs

Ice Packs or Cool Packs: These are great to use after sex if there's a lot of burning and irritation. Make sure you wrap the ice pack in a towel or t-shirt to avoid burns. Use for 10 to 20 minutes or as needed.

Traditional Hot Packs: I always recommend moist heat or hot water bottles but an electric pad would do as well. Make sure to wrap the hot packs to avoid burning yourself. Place the hot pack for 10 to15 minutes and repeat the application as needed. There are many places you can place the packs; it all depends on where the pain is. The following is a list of places that are usually affected by pelvic pain and benefit from heat. You can also try ice and see what works better for you.

1. Vulva (make sure the heat source is wrapped in a towel or t-shirt)
2. Inner thighs
3. Gluteal muscles
4. Lower back, tailbone or sacroiliac joint area
5. Between gluteal muscles on the rectal area

6. Abdominal muscles (great to apply before abdominal rolling)

Portable Cold/Hot Packs: Many of my patients find relief with their hot or cold packs. It always surprises me that such a simple modality can have dramatic effects in reducing pelvic pain and muscle spasms. My patients also love their portable heat and ice pads. These pads can bring comfort and help reduce pain while you are at work or during long plane trips, and can be used everyday to help keep painful muscle spasms at bay. They can be purchased at any pharmacy and are light and easy to put in your purse. Always follow the directions for your portable cold and hot packs.

Castor Oil Packs

Castor oil has been used for medicinal purposes dating back to ancient Egypt. It is derived from the bean of the ricinus communis plant also called palma christi because of its palm-shaped leaves and its miraculous healing properties. Castor oil packs were introduced by Edgar Cayce, the father of modern holistic medicine. Castor oil packs are the external use of castor oil and are commonly used by alternative healers for a variety of conditions and health problems.

Castor oil packs help to promote healing of the tissues and organs underneath the skin. They help increase blood and lymphatic flow, relieve constipation and decrease congestion of abdominal organs. Additionally castor oil packs can improve the autoimmune system, relieve pain from arthritis and tendonitis, and are used to break up scar and abdominal adhesions. For pelvic-pain patients castor oil packs are commonly used to decrease pelvic congestion by improving blood circulation to the abdominal organs. Many women use castor oil packs to break up adhesions after abdominal surgeries. Others use the packs to treat fibroids, ovarian cysts and to improve fertility.

WHAT TO DO:

1. Soak flannel or cotton material in castor oil so that it is thoroughly soaked and saturated but not dripping wet.

2. Place the pack over the affected body part. Cover the castor oil with plastic. Place the hot water bottle or heating pad over the pack. When using a heating pad put in on the medium to high setting. **Do not fall asleep with the heating pad on. Make sure to use a heating pad with an automatic shut-off button.**

3. Leave it on for 45 to 60 minutes. Rest while the pack is in place. This is a great time to meditate and/or practice your reverse Kegels.

4. It is generally recommended for non-acute conditions to use a castor oil pack 3 times per week, every other day. On the fourth week, rest and do not apply a castor oil pack. It is best to consult with your healthcare provider for your specific treatment regimen.

5. After removing the pack, cleanse your skin with a diluted solution of water and baking soda.

6. Store the pack in a covered container in the refrigerator. Each pack may be reused up to 25 to 30 times and can last for 6 months.

WHAT TO WATCH OUT FOR:

1. Castor oil should not be taken internally, as it is a harsh laxative.

2. Castor oil packs should not be applied to broken skin.

3. Castor oil should not be used on C-section or abdominal scars before 6 weeks. Please make sure to consult your doctor before applying a castor oil pack to your scars.

4. Castor oil packs should not be used during pregnancy, breastfeeding, or during menstrual flow.

Chapter Thirteen

"In the midst of movement and chaos,
keep stillness inside of you."
— Deepak Chopra

Chapter 13

BETTER BATHROOM HABITS

As unbelievable as it sounds, something as simple as bad bathroom habits compounded over many years can often be the root cause of pelvic pain and muscle spasms. Many of my patients are surprised to hear that they have been going to the bathroom incorrectly for years and are even more surprised at how much relief they get once they make a few corrections to their basic voiding habits. Often times people are not aware or do not focus their attention when they are in the bathroom, and the results can be prolonged painful flare-ups and overall vulvar irritation. Proper potty posture is one of the simplest and most effective techniques in your toolbox that will have a tremendous impact on your overall healing journey.

Proper Potty Posture

1. Sit with knees above hips, legs wide apart and feet plantar flexed, which means on your toes. For women under five feet tall, use a footstool or book if necessary. Taller women may not need to elevate feet to maintain the above position.

2. Lean forward and place elbows on your thighs. Keep the arch in your back and avoid slumping or rounding the lower back.

3. Gently bulge out your abdominals while simultaneously widening your waist as if to "brace" yourself from a blow to the abdomen.

4. Once you can bulge and brace simultaneously this can be used as a toilet technique, as it will help relax the pelvic floor muscles and facilitate defecation. Doing the "potty posture" takes time but with practice you will master it.

5. Avoid straining. Do not hold your breath. Instead, grunt or groan while bearing down. Play with different sounds such as *ooh*, *ah*, and *shh* which will help further relax your pelvic floor muscles.

Top Bathroom Habits

1. Avoid Constipation. Most individuals who suffer from constipation push and strain to get the stool out. This excessive straining adversely affects your pelvic floor muscles, causing them to be more stressed, leading to increased muscle spasms and pain. **Strategy:** Make sure to get an adequate amount of fiber, drink plenty of water, and always use the "potty posture" as described in the earlier pages of this chapter.

2. Avoid Pushing Urine Out. Most of my patients who suffer from pelvic pain and pelvic floor muscle tightness always complain that they feel as though they can't get the urine out (called feelings of incomplete emptying) or that it takes awhile for the urine stream to start (called hesitancy of urine flow). This makes them push to get the urine out. As stated before, pushing or forcing urination leads to pelvic floor muscle strain which eventually will increase your pelvic pain. **Strategy:** If you are having trouble getting the urine out without pushing, perform quick Kegels and then return to the bathroom later, or try getting up from the toilet, standing for a few minutes, and then sit down again.

3. Avoid Poor Potty Posture. Avoid poor body mechanics and postural alignment such as rounded lower back or slumped upper back while seated on the toilet during defecation. **Strategy:** Use correct "potty posture" to align your spine and internal organs and relax your pelvic floor muscles. This will facilitate elimination without strain or stress on the pelvic floor muscles. Also, remember to never hold your breath with defecation or elimination as this will stress your pelvic floor muscles.

4. Avoid Poor Bladder Health and Habits. Avoid urinating out of habit instead of when a proper urge is present to maintain excellent bladder health. **Strategy:** Normal voiding is 6 to 8 times a day, with a 4 to 5 hour interval. If you do not meet the above criteria, get help in establishing better bladder health. Ask your physical therapist, urologist, internist, or other caregiver to help you get on the right track. Make sure you are also taking in enough water to avoid having highly concentrated urine, a bladder irritant which contributes to an increased urge to urinate.

Tracking Your Bladder and Bowel Health

To bring awareness and to start normalizing your bladder and bowel health, keep track of your voiding and defecation. I have included a voiding diary in Table 13.1 that you can use for tracking your habits as you begin to correct issues that you may not even be aware are contributing to your condition. Once you have filled in your diary, take it to your physical therapist, urologist, or nurse and let them help you reestablish proper habits. In the following chart, ask yourself the following:

1. What is your voiding interval? Is it 15 minutes, 45 minutes, 4 hours, etc?

2. What foods are you eating that could be causing bladder irritation? For a complete guide to foods that cause bladder irritation, consult the fantastic online resource at *www.ic-network.com*.

3. Do you feel like you have to urinate all the time (urgency of urination)? If so, use the following urge-suppression techniques.
    a. Distraction of the mind to delay voiding

    b. Quick flick Kegels, as covered in Part II on page 71.

    c. Diaphragmatic breathing

4. How much water are you drinking during the day? Drink at least 6 to 8 cups of water per day to keep urine diluted. Concentrated urine is highly irritating to the bladder.

Table 13.1: Daily Voiding Diary

PDF version of this table available at http://www.Renew-PT.com

Time of Day	Food Intake	Water Intake (ounces)	Amount Urinated (counted in Mississippis)	Urge Present or Leaking? (Y/N)
6AM				
7AM				
8AM				
9AM				
10AM				
11AM				
12PM				
1PM				
2PM				
3PM				
4PM				
5PM				
6PM				
7PM				
8PM				
9PM				
10PM				
11PM				
12AM				
Overnight				

Chapter Fourteen

"Most of the important things in the world have been accomplished by people who have kept on trying when there seemed to be no hope at all."

- Dale Carnegie

Chapter 14

TRICKS OF THE TRADE

In order to fight back and take control of your pain, you need to have at your disposal a vast arsenal of tools. You could always just take lots of Motrin™ or stronger pain medications to control pain and numb the mind, but at the end of the day these just mask the root causes of pain. My goal is for you to have the tools and food for thought that will help you regain your inner peace, eliminate pain, and give you a better long-term approach for future flare-ups or moments when your pain may reoccur. Some of the techniques in this chapter describe how to use tools that are readily available, such as tennis balls, Thera Canes, and Knobbles. Other techniques I want you to have in your toolkit include electrical stimulation (TENS) and biofeedback technology, both of which you would have to consult your physical therapist or doctor to obtain. I have also included a detailed description of some effective strain-counterstrain techniques that you can do yourself, which are fantastic techniques for releasing spasms and pain in the muscles of your pelvic floor and the muscles that are in close relationship to the PFMs. If you incorporate these trade secrets into your self-healing journey, you can improve your chances of obtaining long-lasting pain relief.

Tennis Ball Massage for Piriformis Release

My patients swear by their tennis balls for pain relief in the lower back and gluteal areas. What I recommend is that they place a tennis ball on the painful body parts and roll it back and forth until the pain starts to dissipate. At first the pain can be excruciating but the longer you do it the better you will feel. Experiment with what works best for you. Sometimes I have my patients just keep the tennis ball stationary on the most painful spot of most pain for 60 to 90 seconds and then have them begin to roll the ball around the painful area. With consistency the result is almost always a reduction in pain and a loosening of painful trigger points.

Common locations for Tennis Ball Massage:

1. Gluteal muscles
2. Upper hip muscles
3. Upper back muscles
4. Sacrum
5. Hip bones
6. On either side of the spine, you can use two tennis balls simultaneously.

TheraCane™

The Thera Cane™ is a great tool for trigger point releases in painful muscles and works great on muscles that are difficult to reach. Place the Thera Cane™ on the painful spot and hold it against the area with consistent pressure for 60 to 90 seconds. Repeat as needed. One of the best resources on the market for the use of the Thera Cane™ is *The Trigger Point Therapy Workbook* by Claire Davies.

Theracane™

Recommended areas for Thera Cane™ placement:

1. Inner thigh muscles

2. Gluteal muscles

3. Lower back muscles including the quadratus lumborum

4. Upper back

5. Abdominal muscles, avoiding artery pulses in the abdominal muscles

Psoas Release with Thera Cane™

Your body has 2 very deep muscles on either side of the lower abdomen called the psoas muscles. These muscles attach from the lower spine to the hip bones, and help flex the hips. The psoas muscles are frequently very painful, in spasm, and irritated in females suffering from pelvic pain.

To find the psoas muscles do the following:

1. Lie on your back with your legs straight out.

2. Go about 2 to 3 inches to the right side of your belly button. Place your fingertips into the area, slowly allowing them to sink into your abdomen and being careful to avoid any feelings of an artery pulse.

3. Lift your right leg straight up and you will feel the psoas pop into your hand. It may take a little practice to get this down but keep trying. Now that you know where the psoas muscle is, place your Thera Cane™ in that spot and slowly press downward into the psoas for 60 to 90 seconds. If you feel any tingling, numbness, or tremendous increase in pain, get off the area and try to relocate the psoas muscle. Switch sides and do the left psoas muscle release.

The Knobble™

The Knobble™ is a smaller version of the Thera Cane™ and is a great tool to use on trigger points. For best results, find the painful spots and press the Knobble™ into the spot for 60 to 90 seconds. The great thing about the Knobble™ is that it easily fits into you purse and can be taken with you to work or when you are away from home on vacation.

Common Areas for the Knobble:

1. Inner thigh

2. Abdominals

3. Gluteal muscles

4. Psoas muscle

5. Low back muscles

6. Upper hip muscles

TENS Unit

Transcutaneous Electrical Stimulation (TENS) is a noninvasive, nonaddictive, drug-free tool that helps many of my patients manage their pelvic pain. You will have to get a prescription from your doctor to get a TENS unit. Prices range from $50 to $1000, so shop wisely. Many times insurance will cover the cost of the units.

How Does It Work?

Soft conductive pads transmit low voltage electrical impulses to areas where the pads are placed. These electrical impulses suppress pain by blocking pain signals before they reach the brain. Pain relief varies among individuals. For some, pain relief is felt immediately while the TENS unit is on. For others, relief continues even after the unit is turned off.

Wearing a TENS unit can bring relief while doing your daily activities. Many of my patients wear a smaller-sized TENS units that can be clipped on their clothes while at work or traveling long distances.

Finding the right placement and setting for your TENS unit is key in reducing pelvic, bladder and lower back pain. Work with your physical therapist to find the right energy pulse setting depending on the exact nature of your condition. Your therapist can also help you with the correct placement of the pads. The large electrodes allow a lot of area to be covered so pad placement does not have to be exact. In the next few pages you will see my most tried and true TENS pad placements that give you relief.

Location of Pads of the TENS Unit

See photos for correct electrode placement.

1. **Along the spine** to the side of pain.

Helps reduce low back pain, hip pain, and general pelvic pain.

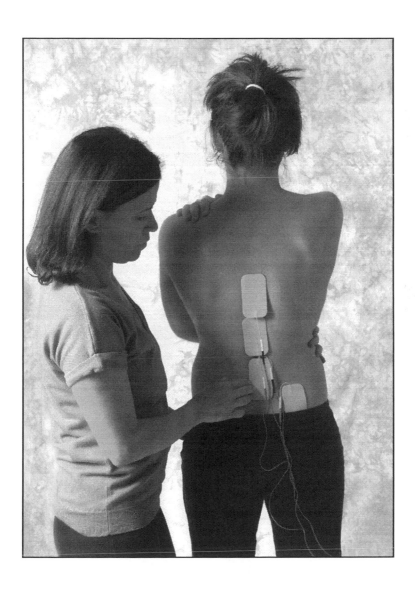

2. **Lower back**

Helps reduce sacral pain, low back pain, hip pain, and pelvic pain. Pads go on either side of the spine in the low back area.

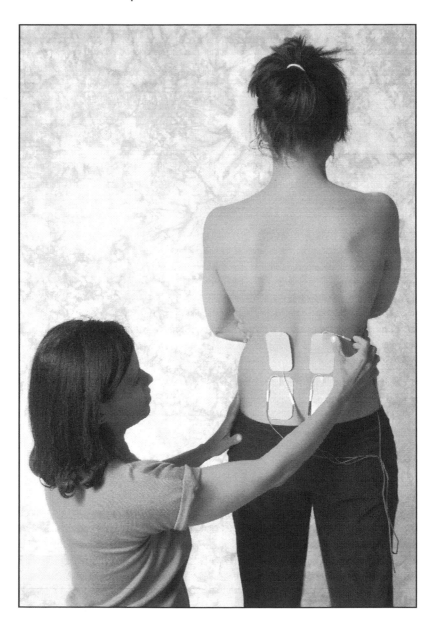

3. **Lower back and gluteal muscles**

Helps reduce low back, pelvic, and gluteal pain, and sciatica.

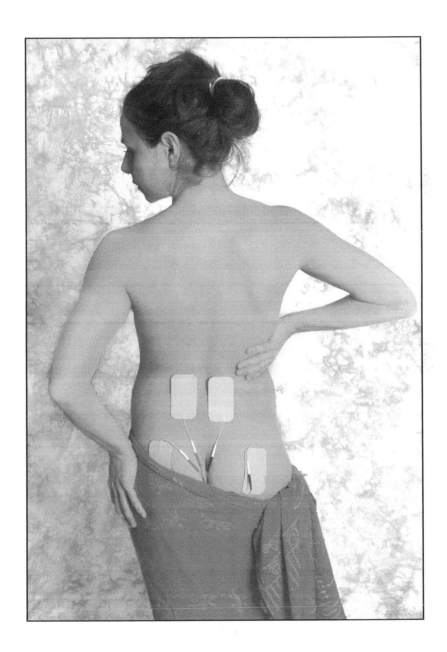

4. Pudendal nerve

Helps reduce pain with pudendal nerve neuropathy and pain with sitting.

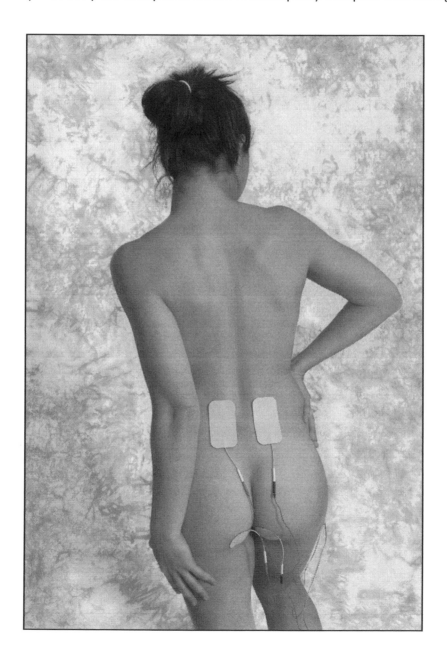

5. **Bladder**

Helps reduce pain with sitting, pain with positional changes, bladder pain, and generalized pelvic pain. Place pads in a semicircle near and around pubic and hip bones.

Biofeedback Technology

Biofeedback technology is a great tool for pelvic floor muscle retraining because it allows you to visualize your PFMs, which are difficult to see. I use biofeedback in conjunction with the various techniques listed throughout this book because it gives me an objective measure and helps me establish a treatment plan for my patient. Biofeedback uses sensors, both externally and/or internally to get electrical readouts from the muscles and how they perform. The units I use in the healing center hook up to a laptop and provide great visuals for my patients so they can see when they are doing Kegels correctly, or downtraining their PFMs correctly. Once they see the readout and feel how the PFMs should be working, it is much easier to repeat the techniques and exercises at home.

The biofeedback also gives me a reading of a patient's resting baseline measured in microvolts, so I can know if their "relaxed state" is truly relaxed.

Usually a pelvic pain patient will have a high resting baseline with the biofeedback of over 2 microvolts. Biofeedback is scientific and allows the patient to understand what it feels like to relax and to let go of the tension in these muscles as they try to lower their baseline.

Biofeedback training might be covered by your health insurance plan. I recommend doing biofeedback with guidance of a physical therapist that can help to cue you. Some facilities do what is called unguided biofeedback, where you are left alone in the room to figure things out for yourself, which I do not recommend. Once you get the basics down with your physical therapist, you can also rent these machines and reeducate your muscles in the privacy of your own home.

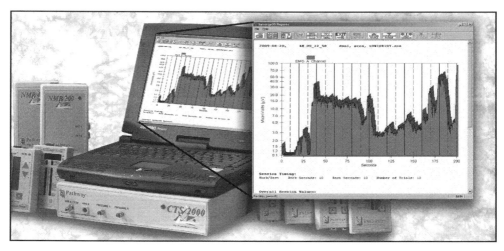

Biofeedback is a great way to get a readout of how your muscles are working together. Through internal and external sensors, the software provides your PFM muscle baseline output in microvolts, helping you visualize while downtraining or uptraining.

Strain-Counterstrain

Strain-counterstrain techniques can have dramatic pain-relieving effects for those suffering from pelvic, hip, and gluteal pain. I have found that when I use these techniques as part of my patients' treatment sessions they often get immediate relief, and have better mobility and improved range of motion in stubborn, tight muscles.

The strain-counterstrain technique was developed by Dr. Lawrence Jones, an osteopathic doctor. It is a gentle and safe technique that passively shortens the affected muscle areas by holding those muscles in a contracted state for 90 seconds. When the muscle is held in this position, it gradually returns to its original resting position and length and is therefore less painful. It's pretty easy to do as part of your self-care as well. These techniques are great to use with a partner but you can also just use them on your own with some modifications. I have included the top two that I think are the easiest to do on yourself and that could give you the most pain relief.

Always grade your pain on a scale of 0 to 10. Grading your pain this way tracks your progress to see if your pain is improving. Remember, it is important to come out of this position slowly and mindfully. Also keep in mind that strain-counterstrain techniques are great to use during your period as they are both external methods.

Obturator Internus Strain-Counterstrain

Obturator internus (OI) pain is very common in woman with vulvodynia. Frequently, pain with deep sexual thrusting can be a result of trigger points or spasms located in this muscle. This muscle is a big culprit of sexual pain as the pudendal nerve travels in its fascia and the pelvic floor muscles also have a connection to this muscle.

WHAT TO DO:

1. Lie on your stomach, find your right sit bone with your right hand and go slightly medial to it, towards the inside of the bone. Press inwards towards the right sit bone and look for painful spots. Here is where the trigger point is commonly found for the OI.

2. While holding the spot with your right hand, bend your right knee to 90 degrees and allow the foot to fall inwards, producing external rotation of the hip. The OI muscle will "pop" into your hand.

3. Hold the spot with the knee bent and rotated for 90 seconds and retest to see if your pain has decreased. Repeat on the left side.

General Pelvic Floor Muscle (Pubococcygeus and Iliococcygeus) Strain-Counterstrain

This strain-counterstrain alleviates overall pelvic floor muscle pain. Symptoms associated with dysfunction in the pelvic floor muscles could be pelvic pain, rectal pain, deep sexual thrusting pain, pubic bone pain, and bladder issues. It is very simple to do and a powerful technique for a generalized pelvic floor muscle release.

WHAT TO DO:

1. To locate this trigger point, palpate internally inside the vagina or find it in the perineum near the sit bones and coccyx/tailbone area.

2. Lie on your back with your hips and knees bent and place a towel under your sacrum and coccyx/tailbone area.

3. Place your right hand over your pubic bone and press the pubic bone with your fingers towards your back, and hold for 90 seconds.

Bulbocavernosus Strain-Counterstrain

The bulbocavernosus is part of the first layer of the pelvic floor muscles. If the bulbocavernosus muscle is in spasms or has trigger points in it there can be pain with initial sexual penetration. If this muscle is in extreme spasms, there might not be any penetration at all. This technique can be extremely helpful before sexual intercourse or as part of your dilator healing program.

WHAT TO DO:

1. Start comfortably in an inclined seated position propped up on some pillows. It's best to remove your underwear for this strain-counterstrain method.

2. Place your index and ring fingers on either side of the clitoris and press your fingers downward towards your perineal body.

3. Place another finger from your other hand over your perineal body and press the perineal body in a superior direction towards your clitoris. You're basically bringing both parts towards each other. Hold this shortened position for 90 seconds. Repeat as necessary.

Proprioceptive Neuromuscular Techniques (PNF)

PNF techniques, short for Proprioceptive Neuromuscular Facilitation isometric techniques, can help release tension in the pelvic floor muscles naturally. The following PNF pattern works particularly well to help maintain a relaxed state in the PFMs.

WHAT TO DO:

1. Lie on your back with your knees bent and aligned with your hips so that your hips and knees form a right angle.

2. Place your hands on the top of your knees, allowing your knees to move outward, as in the photo.

3. As you exhale, press your hands into your knees and your knees into your hands, giving yourself resistance, but not allowing the position to change.

4. The line of force is going to be towards your shoulders, but don't let your hands or legs move.

5. Concentrate on feeling the relaxation of the PFMs and then try to perform a reverse Kegel.

6. Hold for 10 seconds, rest for 10 seconds, repeat 3 times per set, 2 to 3 times per day.

Let's tie it all together now by connecting our physical bodies to our minds by using the techniques in the next chapter, to end the mental chatter that actually contributes to the cycle of pain more than you can imagine.

Chapter Fifteen

"Prosperity is a great teacher;
but adversity a greater teacher."
— William Hazlitt

Chapter 15

MIND/BODY VISUALIZATIONS
AND LIFE STRATEGY TECHNIQUES

Chronic pelvic pain can have devastating effects on a woman's life. The sense of loss and isolation that often accompanies this condition can leave a large hole in your heart and soul. The women that I treat come to their sessions with such sadness that it is difficult for them to hide the demoralizing effects that chronic pelvic pain has on their lives. Many of my patients tell me their partners end up leaving them because they are unable to participate fully in a sexual relationship, causing depression and pessimism to overtake their lives. Many others live in strained relationships with their partners. No matter how you see it, pelvic pain is a difficult condition to live with.

Typical Stories

My patient Harriet, who loved her man very much, couldn't have sex with him anymore because the pain was just too much to bear. In the end, Harriet's boyfriend left her because of the problems with intimacy. The bad part was that Harriet did not want to get involved in a relationship again, which I commonly see in my patients with chronic pain. She's lived her life in isolation and fear that she would never get better again. Every time she meets a man she gets nervous and stresses out because she knows the topic of sex will come up, and she's still not well enough to participate in a sexual relationship. Another patient Lynn, a beautiful young woman, got involved with a much older man because she knew he would not request sex from her. She seemed okay with the relationship but she told me she doesn't really love him. His companionship means a lot to her even if there was no sex, but she was left depressed and pessimistic.

There's also Michelle, a high-powered lawyer who worked so many hours she had "no time" for romance. The long hours kept her safely in a cocoon so she wouldn't have to put herself out there. The stress of Michelle's job would exacerbate her symptoms to the point that when she got home at night she would have to take a pain killer to sleep at night.

Another woman Danelle shows the great length that women will go to have a sexual relationship in spite of their chronic pelvic pain. After Danelle had her baby she could no longer have sex without pain. She experienced a third degree perineal tear during birth and reported feeling that the attending doctor closed her vagina up too tightly, such that her husband now no longer fit into her vagina. She would try to satisfy her husband with oral stimulation, but eventually he became frustrated, angry and resentful because of the lack of sex. Danelle also felt trapped, depressed and became filled with pessimism, feeling that she did not have a choice because she didn't want a divorce.

As you can see in the previous examples, many of my patients who suffer from chronic pain experience an array of emotions that include hopelessness, despair, sadness and catastrophic thinking that contributes to their feelings that they will never get better. These feelings only get worse when the pain is compounded over the years, making them feel out of control. Suffering from chronic pelvic pain can rob you of precious life moments because the pain cycle does not always allow you to participate fully in relationships. Oftentimes, even jobs are affected since many chronic pain sufferers have to miss work.

What I have observed from patients is that if you don't address the mental component of your pain, your condition will create havoc on your mind, soul and body. Although chronic stress does not cause pelvic pain, chronic stress and pessimism can make the pain worse, making you more sensitive to pain and thus causing more flare-ups. I also find it very difficult to treat patients successfully when they are chronically negative and in a state of stress. Many times I have to get them to relax during their treatment sessions before we can even do any treatments. When I incorporate mind-body relaxation techniques into my patients' self-care and home exercise programs, they always do better in the long-term. What I have also noticed is that women who do the best with my treatments are those who are able to defeat negativity by incorporating stress reduction mind-body techniques as part of their healing program.

The Physiology of Stress

Your body undergoes many physiological changes when you become stressed out. The first thing that happens is that your endocrine system reacts by releasing many different types of stress hormones into your bloodstream including adrenaline and cortisol. These hormones awaken you mentally, physically and prepare your body for an emergency response. The body goes through physical changes as well, including increased heart rate, tightening of the muscles, increased sharpness and keenness of the five senses, elevation of blood pressure, increase in perspiration, and shunting of blood from the small muscles to the large muscles of the arms and legs. In addition, your physical strength increases, your reaction time gets faster, and your focus is sharper. These bodily changes prepare you to either fight or flee from a dangerous situation. When real danger is present, stress is a good thing and can motivate you to perform better in life. But when stress is an everyday occurrence it can be detrimental to your health and relationships, eventually clouding your thinking and leading to feelings of being overwhelmed. If you're stressed over a busy schedule, an argument with a friend, a traffic jam, or a mountain of bills, your body reacts just as strongly as if you were facing a life-or-death situation. If you have a lot of responsibilities and worries, your emergency stress response may be "on" most of the time. The more your body's stress system is activated, the easier it is to fall into a pain response or flare-up and the harder it is to shut it off.

Long-term stress can even rewire the brain, leaving you more vulnerable to anxiety and depression. Researchers at the Northwestern University Institute of Neuroscience found that people suffering with chronic back pain, for example, not only demonstrate abnormal brain chemistry, particularly in the emotional center of the brain, but also actual brain shrinkage (*The Journal of Neuroscience,* November, 2004).

For pelvic pain sufferers it is extremely important to manage stress and keep it in check. I have included several techniques and exercises that I use as part of my Renew Program for Women™, helping my patients manage their stress and overcome catastrophic thinking. These stress reduction techniques, meditations, affirmations, and visualizations are easy to do and require no special equipment and can be done anywhere and anytime.

Table15.1: Stress Reduction Techniques

Frequency: Daily

TECHNIQUE
1. Breathing
2. Cardiovascular Stress Reduction
3. Progressive Relaxation with Jacobson's Techniques
4. Positive Thinking vs. Negative Self-Talk
5. Mantras and Meditation
6. Journaling
7. Affirmations
8. Keep It Simple – Stop Taking on Too Much
9. Join a Self-Help Group
10. Gratitude Training – Rock and Walk
11. The Present Moment – Staying in the Power of Now
12. Creative Visualizations

Breathing

Focusing on your breathing can have tremendous benefits for your overall stress level. It also helps you to quiet your mind and centers your attention on the present moment. Most people don't take the time to focus on their breathing during the course of the day, but this powerful yet simple exercise can help you release tension, stress, and anxiety.

WHAT TO DO:

1. Sit in cross-legged position, stand or lie down in a relaxed comfortable position.

2. Slowly inhale through your nose, counting to 5 in your head.

3. Exhale from your mouth, counting to 10 in your head. The exhale counting depends on your comfort. Some women may find that exhaling for 10 seconds is too long and causes anxiety or shortness of breath.

TIPS:

1. As you breathe, let your lower abdomen expand outward, keeping your shoulders quiet and low. Avoid raising your shoulders as you inhale and exhale. Breathing this way enhances relaxation and it's a natural way to breathe. Breathing like this also helps fill your lungs more fully with fresh air and helps to release old stagnant air.

2. Repeat several times a day for 5 to10 minutes. Great to do at work, during stressful situations, and while meditating.

3. To release more tension, exhale so the air comes out like a whisper by pursing lips. This kind of breathing is done in many yoga classes.

4. Focus on releasing your stress in your exhale, attaching your stress to your breath as it leaves your body.

Cardiovascular Stress Reduction

Cardiovascular exercise for at least 30 minutes a day is a great stress buster and it also helps to release natural endorphins that help relieve pain. The one exercise that anyone can do is walking which is why I always recommend a walking program to release stress.

WHAT TO DO:

1. Walk during your lunch hour instead of having lunch at your desk. Follow your lunch-time walk with the workplace stretches listed in Chapter 7 of this book.

2. Take an evening walk after dinner instead of sitting in front of your computer or sitting to watch TV.

3. Join a gym and walk on the treadmill when it's cold outside. You can also do a walking program in a mall when it's cold outside.

4. Combine your walking with your gratitude meditation as well, which I will describe later in this chapter. This is a really positive way to build a permanent change to your overall thought patterns.

5. As an alternative to walking, try stationary biking and then see how you feel. Make sure you wear padded bike pants. Be careful of the bikes, though, because they can add too much pressure on the perineum and pelvic floor muscles.

Progressive Relaxation with Jacobson's Techniques

Progressive muscle relaxation was developed by Dr. Edmund Jacobson more than 50 years ago. Dr. Jacobson discovered through his work with his patients that a muscle could be relaxed by first voluntarily tensing it for a few seconds. This voluntary contraction and subsequent muscle relaxation of various body areas produces a deep state of relaxation. Dr. Jacobson found that this technique of progressive relaxation was capable of relieving a variety of conditions, from high blood pressure to ulcerative colitis, to overall pain.

GENERAL GUIDELINES:

This relaxation technique requires that you alternately tense and relax your muscles. Try to practice this relaxation at the same time each day for 15 to 30 minutes. Find a comfortable position such as supported incline sitting or laying down. Start with the breathing techniques described above for 5 to 10 minutes. The best way to start is to work with groups of muscles in the following sequence but you can also develop a system that works for you.

Basic Jacobson Contract Relax Sequence
WHAT TO DO:

1. Contract the right arm for 10 seconds and then relax your right arm for 15 to 20 seconds. Do the same for left arm.

2. Contract both shoulders for 10 seconds and then relax your shoulders for 15 to 20 seconds.

3. Contract your neck muscles for 10 seconds and then relax your neck muscles for 15 to 20 seconds.

4. Contract your lips and eyes by closing them tightly for 10 seconds and then relax your lips and eyes for 15 to 20 seconds.

5. Contract whole right leg including toes and ankle tightly for 10 seconds and then relax your whole right leg for 15 to 20 seconds. Do the same for the left leg.

6. This is a basic sequence but you can separate out the body parts and tense and relax as many body parts as you want. The more body parts you individually contract and relax the longer this relaxation will take.

Positive Thinking vs. Negative Self-Talk

Oftentimes, my patients can be their own worst enemies. Self-sabotaging thoughts in the form of negative self-talk prevent them from doing the things they need to do to get better. Sometimes the self-sabotaging thoughts are even subconscious, and my patients don't even realize they are doing it habitually until I point it out to them. These women are filled with thoughts like "I'll never get better," "sex will always hurt," and "this is the best I will ever feel."

I am a firm believer that the body will follow your mind. What you think is what you are. The way we talk to ourselves can make a situation sunny and bright or can take the same situation and make it dark, cloudy and gloomy. Pay attention to the story that your thoughts are creating about your life. Acknowledge your thoughts, but don't always take them as gospel. You can change your entire life by first changing your negative self-talk into more positive, focused and optimistic thought patterns.

Mantras and Meditation

I give my patients mantras to get them through the day. A mantra is a repeated word, syllable, phrase, or sound that can help you relax during times of stress or as a precursor to your stretching, strengthening or dilator work. Saying a mantra during meditation or at various times throughout the day will help quiet your mind and bring inner peace to you. The most basic mantra is OM. This mantra can be repeated slowly for 3 to 5 minutes and it brings a calming feeling to your entire body. Allow the syllable or syllables of your mantra to resonate slowly inside your head and body like a bell, using it to clear out the "thought clutter" that often prevents us from staying in the moment. The main objective is to quiet down negative thoughts to make room for positive thoughts to sprout into your consciousness. Remember, you must believe in your mantra, and then your body will follow. I like to have my patients meditate for 3 to 5 minutes while quietly repeating their mantra. This meditation technique with mantras has been shown to lower cholesterol, reduce stress, pain, and blood pressure, and improve heart function.

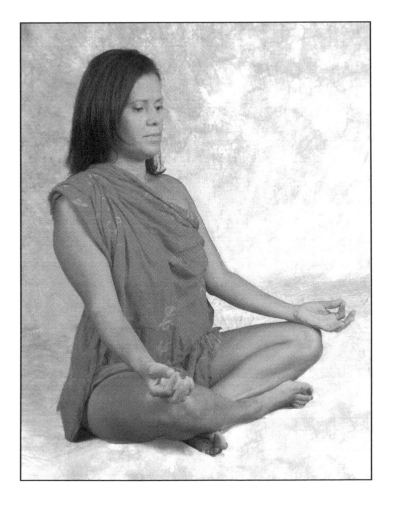

WHAT TO DO:

1. Sit or lie down, usually with your eyes closed.

2. Focus on deep diaphragmatic breathing for 5 to 10 breaths as you slow down your mind. Many of my patients report holding their breath or breathing shallowly when they experience pain, which limits oxygen to the tissues and results in more pain. You must do the opposite during your meditation.

3. Begin repeating your mantra with conviction, allowing it to permeate into your being.

4. After 3 to 5 minutes, resume diaphragmatic breathing and then after you feel comfortable, repeat the mantra or try a different one.

Mantra Samples

Om Shanti Om

I-Am-Pain-Free

I-Am-Healed

Journaling

I often tell my patients to keep a journal of their journeys up to the present moment. I tell them to write down the stories of their pain as they perceive it. Sometimes the pain is a result of a traumatic incident from childhood. I had a patient tell me she had her pain since she fell off a trampoline as a youngster. Other patients don't tell me but I get a sense that their pain is the result of sexual abuse. Oftentimes they don't completely remember what happened but they feel that their body's response has been one of "closing down" in an effort to protect itself. Still other patients' pain journeys are the result of giving birth to their children and not getting the proper care and encouragement to get their bodies back. Other new moms carry a sense of shame because they had

C-sections instead of natural births, and thus develop pain as it relates to their low self-esteem surrounding their birth experience.

Whatever the story of your pain may be, I encourage my patients to write it down and track their feelings as they journey forward with The Renew Program For Women™ Once you have it written down, I often suggest my patients to perform a ceremony where they burn or shred their story and release the past from their body and mind. I first did this after a painful, late-stage miscarriage. My husband and I were filled with pain and anguish, and thought we could not move forward. We ended up journeying to the mountains in Spain where we burned the printouts of the sonograms of our baby, releasing the past from our psyches. It was hard to do but it ended up being a wonderful experience that brought us tremendous feelings of peace and acceptance, and cleared out the past. Once you let go of the mental burden of your own pain story, you can free your consciousness to spring forward to positive thoughts and allow the healing energy of the universe to flow once again through your body and mind.

Affirmations

It is always remarkable to me how powerful your words can be in shaping your actions and your life. I am a firm believer that your body will follow what you say you are. So if you are a person who suffers from chronic pain, you might not realize that what you say could be perpetuating your suffering as much as your thoughts. As you go through your day, try to see yourself from the outside and actually listen to the words you use to describe yourself and your various situations in your life, from your job, to your relationships, to your perception of your own existence. You might find that you are actually saying out loud that you won't get better, you are destined to be in pain, or that it is your fate to be afflicted.

By using affirmations to change your spoken words about your perceived life situations, you can create powerful forces of change that your body will eventually follow. I like to have my patients write down their affirmations and say them in the mirror while looking themselves in the eye. Repeat them every morning before brushing your teeth and every evening before going to bed, and you will find your words will change your life. Say them with conviction and the changes you desire will come more quickly. I always recommend my patients read Louise Hay's great book, *You Can Heal Your Life*, to get a more in-depth analysis of the power of affirmations. I have included here some great affirmations for women with pelvic pain, but it is also great if you write some of your own as well. Remember to write your affirmations in the present tense with words like "I am," or "I have", so your mind can tell your body that these are states of life that you already are in, not some distant place where you hope to be in the future.

Table 15.2: Affirmations for Pelvic Pain

AFFIRMATION
1. I am healed.
2. I am having great and pain-free sex with my partner.
3. I have supple, soft and pain-free pelvic floor muscles.
4. I am surrounded by love.
5. I am in a loving and satisfying relationship.
6. I have a beautiful baby who came to me as a result of a beautiful birth.

Keep It Simple: Stop Taking on Too Much

Are you taking on too much work or find yourself overscheduled? Are you not sure how to say *no* to other people's demands on your time? If the answer is *yes*, than you can put yourself in a state of chronic stress and you habitually will tend to take on more than you can handle. Do you find you are constantly putting yourself last on your own list? If this is the case you might be subconsciously sabotaging your healing and causing yourself undue stress, tension and pressure.

If you are constantly telling yourself you just don't have time to do your Renew Program For Women™ healing techniques, then you have to break the cycle of taking on too much. If you have to, schedule time for yourself during the day and in the mornings and evenings. Even 15 minutes during the day to do a quick mediation, breathing, mantra, and workplace stretching program will work wonders for your body, mind, and soul. You will also find that once you begin to carve out time for yourself, it becomes easier to keep on doing it because your body and your mind will gravitate to the positive way it makes you feel.

Tips for Keeping It Simple and Not Taking on Too Much

1. Say no to family and friends if it puts you under stress.

2. Make sure that your work schedule does not interfere with your healing work.

3. Space out your social calendar so that you have ME time.

4. Do something that brings you joy and happiness everyday, even if it is as simple as looking at flowers for 5 minutes.

5. Surround yourself with positive energy and avoid being around negative people.

Join a Self-Help Group

I find that the women that do the best in my practice have someone to talk to about their emotional pain. Many of my patients tell me they feel better and less stressed after being surrounded by women who have the same problems as they do. They also tell me that having a sex therapist or psychoanalyst to talk to can be healing, helpful and keeps them positive.

TIPS:

1. Join a self-help group and keep with it for several months.

2. Get a life-coach.

3. See a psychotherapist or a sex therapist for your emotional pain.

4. If there are no groups near you, then a start one yourself or join an Internet blog.

5. Ask your physical therapist if she could help you arrange a self-help group with other patients.

Gratitude Training - Rock and Walk

When I first saw *The Secret* by Rhonda Byrnes I was captured by the part in the DVD when they mentioned having an "Attitude of Gratitude." Another great source for gratitude training is Deepak Chopra, who talks about gratitude and how it needs to be the foundation of your overall outlook. I constantly find that my patients come to me and are so focused on their pain and how it pervades their whole life that it is the only thing on their minds. I always tell them, although they often look at me like I am crazy at first, that they need to think about all of the things they are grateful for instead. I tell them that in order to get on the road to healing, they have to first focus on things that are positive in their lives instead of focusing only on the pain and what they don't have.

Gratitude Rocks

When my patients come to me on their first visit I give them a gratitude rock. This rock is to remind them of the beauty, love and joy that they currently have in their lives.

WHAT TO DO:

1. Find a rock small enough that you can carry with you everyday. I carry mine in my pocket or purse. I collect rocks from the ocean or streams because they are smooth and have all of the rough and symbolically "painful edges" smoothed off by the power of water. I let my patients pick a rock that captures their eye.

2. When you are having a hard day and a pain flare-up, touch your rock and repeat to yourself: "I am grateful today for _____." Think about your statement and feel it. Feel the joy, happiness and elation around your statement. Send these feelings to all your cells, all body parts and muscles.

3. Put the rock next to your bed, and when you wake up, roll up and sit on the edge of your bed. Take your rock in your hand and think about something you are grateful for. Set the tone for your day as one of gratitude, one in which your pain and negativity, if it comes, will only be a fleeting part of your day.

4. Remember that the universe will not give more than you can bear, so stay grateful for things as simple as having enough air to breathe, and you will have a powerful transformational effect on your existence.

Gratitude Walks

As part of your cardiovascular training, incorporate gratitude into your walking program. Be conscious of how your thoughts are taking up space in your mind while you are walking, and make sure to take notice of the beauty around you. If you are walking in the park, take notice of birds, flowers, kids playing, the sunlight shining through the trees, or any other visuals or sounds that should make you feel grateful. Instead of thinking about how much you hate your boss or how much pain you are in, think about how grateful you are to be working at all, and how grateful you are to be on the road to healing, even if you are currently only making the smallest of steps forward in your program. The momentum will build and you will be amazed at the results.

The Present Moment - Staying in the Power of Now

Misery, stress and unhappiness are usually caused by thinking about events that are in the future or in the past. I find that when my patients stay present "in the now" they have less stress and anxiety. A personal favorite is Eckhart Tolle, a great author and lecturer who has written many books including a wonderful book called the *Power of Now*. I recommend this book to my patients, and they tell me they now understand how the constant flurry of activity that occurs in their minds affects their health and overall outlook. It is not difficult to be in the present but you must make an effort to be in the now.

Tolle talks at length about how the mind creates "the story of me," and how your ego tries to interpret events and actions in your life within this context. So if your mind has created a story of me that is one of perpetual pain, then your mind and ego will seek out events and people and interpretations of what has happened to you to keep going with this story. Once you let go of the past and the future, which are only creations of the mind, you can embrace the present moment, which you will find is actually quite manageable and one in which you can make conscious decisions to move forward down the path to your ultimate healing.

TIPS:

1. When thinking about future events or past events bring your mind to the present moment and focus your energy on your current breath. You can acknowledge your thoughts and thank your brain for trying to interpret every perception in the context of "the story of me," but let your mind know that you are going to focus on the present moment right now and enjoy it without interpretation.

2. Get a copy of Eckhart Tolle's book, *The Power of Now*, and read it at least 2 times.

Creative Visualizations

As discussed earlier, you are what you think and say you are, so be careful because the universe will lovingly give you what you think and declare you are. So why not start by thinking and visualizing yourself well, free from excess mental chatter, happy, and pain-free. Creative visualization is a great tool to use to reduce stress related to your painful condition. It's quite easy to do and can consist of almost any visualization. Below are 2 examples I have found that work great for my patients.

The Mirrored Hallway

Several times a day, whenever you are able, take a moment for a mental break and try the mirrored hallway visualization exercise. Repeat the exercise at least once per day for 2 to 4 weeks and track your progress. You should begin to see just how powerful your mind can be in keeping you in a state of pain if you let it, even subconsciously keeping you from declaring that you are better each day.

WHAT TO DO:

1. This exercise can be done sitting or lying down. I like to do this on the subway on my way home.

2. Close your eyes and focus on your breathing for 5 breaths. Focus on slowing down your breathing. Release the thoughts of the day up until that point, inhale through the nose and exhale through the mouth. Don't think about the future or the past.

3. Imagine the lights are being turned on and you find yourself in a short 6 to 8 foot hallway with a door on one end. You are just entering the hallway so the door is at the other end of the hallway.

4. You then notice that there are floor to ceiling mirrors on both sides of the hallway. On the left, see yourself or your situation, allowing your reflection

to be your state of pain, your misery, your negative outlook, anything in life which you wish to overcome.

5. Then look to the right and allow your reflection to be the exact opposite from the left. See yourself in a pain-free state, happy, filled with positive thoughts, having overcome that which your mind tells you cannot overcome. Focus and remember how good you will feel since you have overcome your pain.

6. Then turn back to the left mirror, notice that there is a large wooden staff in the corner of the hallway. Take the staff and smash the mirror on the left in one forceful blow, bringing your mind into that moment, telling your mind that you will not tolerate these reflections to exist any longer.

7. Focus back on the right, and then walk through the hall seeing your reflection, open the door and continue on your journey as a pain-free person.

Mental Suds Visualization

I like to use this visualization as a gauge to help me get a sense of how many thoughts are actually "on my mind." At first you will find how amazingly filled your mind is even when you think you are in the moment. I often use this visualization as I prepare to do a meditation and mantra to calm down my mind.

WHAT TO DO:

1. Sit comfortably, with your eyes closed, with your focus slightly upward towards your third eye. Your third eye is the area above your nose and in between your eyebrows.

2. Allow the thoughts in your head to flow freely into this area of focus. Don't worry if the thoughts are good or bad, simply take notice of them as they cross your focus.

3. As each thought passes into your gaze, place it into a bubble and allow it to float in your perception. Don't let it float away, but keep it within your gaze.

4. Repeat this for each thought that is currently "on your mind." You may find in a short while that all of the bubbles you have created have made what I call "mental suds," where the bubbles are so close together that they look like suds in a bubble bath. If this is the case, don't worry; you have just created a mental picture of what is whizzing through your mind at the present moment.

5. Make an effort to pop bubbles in your field of view, releasing the thoughts contained in each bubble which are not important to your present moment.

6. Try to pop all the bubbles that relate to your past or to things you have to do or that relate to relationships and how you need to talk to this person or that person, or how you are always going to be in pain, etc. Leave just a couple of bubbles in your field of view, maybe one bubble filled with a thought about your breath and how it can heal you, and maybe another bubble filled with a thought about something you are grateful for, and maybe one bubble with a thought about how great it is to be pain-free.

Conclusion

You've done it! You've gone all the way through my book. If this is your first read, go back and begin to absorb the nuances as you experiment with crafting your program from your new sets of tools. Armed with information and determination, embark on your journey to relieving your pain and don't look back.

Remember to keep on track by checking out my website, *www.Renew-PT.com*. I am always adding new material to my great site and invite you to get involved in spreading the word to women who have suffered too long.

Appendix, Glossary Bibliography, and Index

*"Keep your thoughts positive, thoughts become your words.
Keep you words positive, words become your behaviors. Keep
your behaviors positive, behaviors become your habits.
Keep your habits positive, habits become your values. Keep
your values positive, values become your destiny."*

—Gandhi

Appendices

Appendix 1: Resources

Renew Physical Therapy Website. *www.Renew-PT.com*. My website has free information, blank PDFs of charts for your pain mapping, pain journaling, DRA testing, Q-tip test, voiding diary, and other important tools.

American College of Obstetricians and Gynecologists. *www.acog.org*.

American Physical Therapy Association. 1-800-999-APTA. Physical therapy for the pelvic floor- select women's health. *www.APTA.org*.

The Business of Being Born. Great information for all women planning to have a baby. *www.thebusinessofbeingborn.com*.

Dilator Sets. Available on this site. *www.vaginismus.com*.

Endometriosis Association. *www.endometriosisassn.org*.

Herbal and Flower Products. For vaginal steams and penal washes. *www.mountainroseherbs.com*.

Holly Herman & Kathe Wallace. Best teachers in pelvic floor rehab. Call to get a recommendation for a pelvic floor rehab specialist. Telephone: 206-724-7888.

www.pelvicrehab.com.

Menopause Society of North America. *www.menopause.org*

Interstitial Cystitis Network. *www.IC-network.org.*

International Society for the Study of Vulvovaginal Disease. *www.issvd.org.*

IPPS: The International Pelvic Pain Society. *www.PelvicPain.org.*

Midwives Alliance of North America. *www.mana.org.*

My Best Birth. Ricki Lake and Abby Epstein's great resource for women. *www.mybestbirth.com.*

National Fibromyalgia Association. *www.fmaware.org.*

NVA: National Vulvodynia Association. *www.NVA.org.*

Vulvodynia Online Resource. *www.vulvodynia.com.*

Water Based Lubricant. *www.slipperystufflubes.com.*

Appendix 2: The Female Body Musculature

deltoid

pectoralis major

biceps brachii

external oblique

rectus abdominus

linea alba

adductors
(inner thigh muscles)

abductors
(outer thigh muscles)

sartorius

quadriceps

tibialis anterior

Female Anatomy – FRONT VIEW

deltoid

trapezius
(rhomboid major/minor
are deep to trapezius)

latissimus dorsi
(the erector spinae are deep
to the latissimus dorsi)

quadratus lumborum
(deep to the latissimus
dorsi muscle)

gluteus medius

gluteus maximus
(piriformis is deep to
the gluteus maximus)

hamstrings

gastrocnemius
(calf muscles)

soleus

Female Anatomy – BACK VIEW

Glossary

Adhesions. Fibrous bands that form between tissues and organs as a result of the healing process that occurs after surgical procedures, inflammation, trauma or infection.

Alcock's Canal. A structure within the pelvis through which the pudendal nerve, internal pudendal artery and internal pudendal veins travel. This structure is like a canal formed by the obturator internus fascia.

Anismus. A malfunction of the external anal sphincter and puborectalis (part of the PFM) muscle during defecation. Failure of these muscles to relax during defecation causes obstructed defecation and constipation.

Bartholin's Glands. Glands located to the left and right of the vaginal opening that secrete mucus to provide vaginal lubrication.

Biofeedback. Biofeedback training is a nonmedical treatment that helps people improve their health by taking conscious control of their muscles using real-time body signals. Physical therapists use biofeedback to help retrain the pelvic floor muscles.

Cesarean Section (C-Section). A Cesarean section is a major abdominal surgery in which incisions are made through the mother's abdomen and uterus to deliver her child.

Chakra. Chakras are force centers that are believed to pulsate subtle energy. Seven major chakras are believed to exist within the body.

Chronic Pelvic Pain. A pelvic pain condition that persists for longer than three months. It is poorly understood and many times requires a multidisciplinary approach for successful treatment.

Coccyxdynia or Coccygodynia. Pain in the area of the tailbone and its associated structures.

Connective Tissue Rolling. A type of massage that is superficial in nature and can be performed on any part of the body, including but not limited to, the abdomen, thighs, buttocks and lower back.

Dilator. A medical instrument used to stretch and expand the vaginal opening. Dilators are also used for intravaginal and intrarectal massage of the pelvic floor muscles. Many times, dilators are also used for trigger point release therapy.

Dyspareunia. Painful sexual intercourse which can occur for many reasons including medical or psychological. Dyspareunia is almost always reported by women, but this problem can also occur in men.

Episiotomy. An episiotomy is a surgical incision made at the perineum to enlarge the vagina. This incision can be midline or medial-lateral. It is a common cause of sexual pain and can cause scar tissue in the perineum.

Fascia. Fascia is the soft tissue glue that holds the body together. It permeates the entire body, surrounding muscles, organs, nerves, blood vessels and other visceral structures. Fascia helps maintain structural integrity, provides support and protection, and acts as a shock absorber.

Fibromyalgia. A medical disorder that causes widespread body pain exacerbated by gentle touch. Additional symptoms include fatigue, sleep disturbance, and joint stiffness. This condition can also affect the respiratory, digestive and other body systems.

Hart's Line. The edge of the vulvar vestibule frequently examined for pain. The Q-tip test is the gold standard for determining abnormalities and pain in this area.

Hymenectomy. A surgical operation to remove the hymen.

Incontinence. Any involuntary leakage or loss of urine.

Interstitial Cystitis. Interstitial cystitis/painful bladder syndrome (IC/PBS) is a bladder disease characterized by painful urination, urinary frequency and urgency, and pressure in the bladder and/or pelvis. IC can also cause spasms and trigger points in the pelvic floor muscles.

Intra-Abdominal Pressure. Pressure within the abdominal cavity.

Kegel. An exercise named after Dr. Arnold Kegel that consists of contracting and relaxing the pelvic floor muscles.

L1-L5. L1 through L5 represent the five lumbar spinal vertebrae. The lumbar vertebrae are found between the thoracic and sacral vertebrae in the spinal column. Many times, women with pelvic pain will have some kind of associated dysfunction with L5 and the lumbar spine.

Labia. The labia majora are the outer vaginal lips and are composed mostly of skin and adipose (fat) tissue. Protection is their main function. The labia minora are the inner vaginal lips on either side of the vaginal opening. The clitoris is the area where labia minora meet superiorly.

Laparoscopic Procedure. Surgical operations commonly performed within the abdominal or pelvic cavities using small keyhole-size incisions.

Levator Ani Muscles. The muscles that make up the pelvic floor.

Levator Ani Spasms. Involuntary contractions of the pelvic floor muscles that can lead to pain with sexual intercourse, sitting or other simple daily activities.

Levator Ani Syndrome. Consists of pain, pressure, discomfort or deep dull ache in the vagina and rectum, including the sacrum and coccyx. Levator ani syndrome can also cause burning or radiating pain into the thighs and buttocks. Pain with sitting and defecation are common complaints. Many times the pelvic floor muscles are in spasms and have multiple trigger points in them.

Lichen Sclerosus. An uncommon disease which may cause white patches or scarring on and around genital skin.

Marinoff Scale. A scale that quantifies pain as it relates to sexual intercourse.

Mons Pubis. It is the fatty tissue lying above the pubic bone of adult women.

Muscle Spindles. These are sensory receptors located within the belly of a muscle that detect changes in the length of the muscle fiber. This detection plays an important role in regulating muscle contraction. This information also helps the brain to determine the position of the body.

Muscle Golgi Tendon Apparatus. The Golgi tendon organ is a proprioceptive sensory receptor located at the insertion of skeletal muscle fibers. This receptor monitors tension in the muscles. If there is excessive tension, the Golgi tendon will send a message that tells the muscle to relax.

Myomectomy. Refers to the surgical removal of uterine fibroids.

Neuropathic Pain. Neuropathic pain is not related to the activation of pain receptor cells in any part of the body. This type of pain is produced by a change or injury to neurological structure or function of the tissue.

Obturator Internus Muscle. The obturator internus muscle is found within the pelvis, and within the hip-joint. This muscle helps to externally rotate the leg, extended thigh and abduct flexed leg thigh. It also helps to stabilize femoral head in the acetabulum. This muscle can be accessed through the vagina and frequently can have spasms and trigger points causing sexual pain.

Pelvic Floor Muscle Dysfunction. Abnormal or impaired function of the pelvic floor muscles.

Pelvic Floor Muscle Hypertonicity. Muscular hypertonicity is a disorder in which muscles continually receive a message to tighten and to contract. This causes excessive stiffness or tightness and interferes with their normal function.

Pelvic Floor Muscle Incoordination. A lack of normal and harmonious muscle action in the pelvic floor muscles.

Pelvic Floor Muscle Spasm. Involuntary contraction of a pelvic floor muscle.

Pelvic Girdle. The muscles, bones and ligaments of the pelvic and hip region.

Pelvic Release. A lengthening release of the pelvic floor muscles that can be performed with either inhalation or exhalation.

Perineal Body. The central area between the rectum and the vagina in the perineum. It is also the area where most of the pelvic floor muscles are attached.

Perineal Tearing. Tears to the perineum (the area between the genitalia and anus) that can cause damage to the anal sphincter causing fecal incontinence, urgency, pain during intercourse or other problems.

Perineal Tears in Degrees. Tears are rated from 1st to 4th Degree. 1st Degree is tearing of the vaginal mucosa skin at or around the perineal body. 2nd Degree is tearing vaginal mucosa and submucosa through the pelvic floor muscles. 3rd Degree is tearing of the 1st and 2nd Degree tissues and the external sphincter. 4th Degree is all of the above levels of tearing plus the internal sphincter and the lining of the rectum.

Perineum. The diamond-shaped area between the legs that houses muscles and rectum, and in females, includes the vagina. This can also refer to both the superficial or deep structures in this region.

Piriformis Syndrome. A disorder that occurs when the sciatic nerve is compressed, pinched or irritated by the piriformis muscle. This compression can cause pain, tingling and numbness in the buttocks and along the sciatic nerve path.

Prolapse. This term is used for organs that protrude through the vagina. This condition makes the organ drop into the vagina causing pelvic floor muscle weakness. The uterus, rectum, bladder or urthrea can prolapse into the vagina.

Pubic Bone. This bone forms the anterior aspect of the pelvis and hip bones.

Pudendal Neuralgia or Pudendal Nerve Entrapment. Pudendal nerve entrapment (PNE) is a source of chronic pain in which the pudendal nerve is entrapped or compressed. Pain increases with sitting and can include sensations such as stabbing, burning, numbness into the labias, hip muscles and pelvic floor muscles.

Resting Baseline of the Pelvic Floor Muscles. It is the biofeedback readout that reports the activity of the muscles while a person is at rest. Normally, most individuals have low resting baselines; however, women suffering from sexual pain usually have elevated resting baselines.

S2-S5. S2 through S5 are vertebraes of the sacral spine. The sacral spine is below the lumbar spine and is located at the base of the spine.

Sacroiliac Joint (SI Joint). This is the joint between the sacrum and the ilium hip bone joined by ligaments. It is a strong, weight-bearing joint that can generate extreme discomfort for women with chronic pelvic pain.

Sacrum. The sacrum is a triangular bone at the base of the spine where it is inserted like a wedge between the two hip bones. Its upper edge connects to the last lumbar vertebra, and its bottom connects with the coccyx (tailbone). The sacral nerves exit through small holes in the sacrum.

Scar. A scar is part of the natural healing process of wound repair in the skin and other tissues of the body.

Strain-Counterstrain. A technique invented by Dr. Lawrence Jones, where muscles are put in a position of maximum contraction for 90 seconds, allowing the muscle to rest. This technique relieves pain and results in better muscle function.

Tendinous Arch of the Levator Ani. A thickened portion of the obturator fascia where some of the levator ani muscles originate. This fascia can be painful to the touch. Let an experienced PT show you how to correctly release this fascia.

Tension Release Breathing (TRB). A breathing technique coined by author Isa Herrera using mind/body connection to release pain and tension of a painful muscle. The individual inhales into the painful body part while thinking about collecting her pain while inhaling. Then the individual exhales and visualizes the pain leaving her body. This type of breathing should be performed for 5 breaths.

Urgency or Frequency of Urination. Frequent urination or urgency of urination without an increase in the total urine held in the bladder. This condition may result from infections, a small bladder capacity, other structural abnormalities, from food irritants, or trigger points.

Vaginismus. A condition in which the pelvic floor muscles go into spasms or tense suddenly, making penetration impossible. Women who suffer from this condition experience difficulty or pain with sexual relations, problems with inserting tampons, or penetration involved with gynecological examinations. This condition can be a result of an involuntary muscular reflex.

Vestibulitis. An irritation of the vulva. Also called vestibular vulvodynia.

Vestibulectomy. Surgical removal of extremely painful tissue of the vaginal vestibule.

Vulva. The external female genitalia.

Vulvar Biopsy. A biopsy performed under local anesthesia to obtain a small sample of vulvar epithelium for examination.

Vulvar Vestibulitis. Inflammation and pain of the vulvar vestibule that leads to painful sexual intercourse.

Vulvodynia, Provoked. A type of vulvodynia that occurs with direct contact with the vulva.

Vulvodynia, Unprovoked. A type of vulvodynia that causes vulvar pain, burning, and discomfort without direct contact to the vulva area.

Bibliography

Abbott J. (2009). Gynecological indications for the use of botulinum toxin in women with chronic pelvic pain. Toxicon. 2009 Oct; 54(5):647-53. Epub 2009 Mar 3.

Abbott, J., Jarvis, S., Lyons, S., Thomson, A., & Vancaille, T. (2006). Botulinum toxin type A for chronic pain and pelvic floor spasm in women: a randomized controlled trial. Obstetrics & Gynecology, 108(4), 915-923.

Abraham, K. (2002). A special update on chronic pelvic pain from the conference: Chronic pelvic pain: Pathogenic mechanisms, treatment, innovations, and research implications. Journal of the Section on Women's Health, 26(3), 9-12.

Albert, H., Godskesen, M., Westergaard, J. (1999). Evaluation of clinical tests used in classification procedures in pregnancy-related pelvic joint pain. European Spine Journal, 9(2) 161-166.

Arvigo, Rosita, and Epstein, Nadine. (2001). Rainforest Remedies: The Maya Way to Heal Your Body & Replenish Your Soul. New York, New York: Harper Collins Publishers.

Barral, Jean-Pierre. (2007). Visceral Manipulation II (Revised Edtion). Seattle WA: Eastland Press.

Barral, Jean-Pierre and Mercier, Pierre. (2005). Visceral Manipulation, Revised Edition. Seattle, Washington: Eastland Press.

Barral, Jean-Pierre, and Kuchera, Michael L. (2007). Visceral and Obstetric Osteopathy. Edinburgh, England: Churchill Livingstone.

Barral, Jean-Pierre, DO, Wetzler, Gail, RPT, Ahern, Dee, RPT, Grant, Lisa Brady, DC. (2005). Visceral Manipulation: Abdomen 2 Study Guide. West Palm Beach, FL: The Barral Institute.

Barral, Jean-Pierre, DO, Wetzler, Gail, RPT. (2005). Visceral Manipulation: Abdomen 1 Study Guide. West Palm Beach, Florida: The Barral Institute.

Barral, Jean-Pierre. (1993). Urogenital Manipulation. Seattle, WA: Eastland Press.

Bergeron, S., et al. (2001). Vulvar Vestibular Syndrome: Reliability of diagnosis and evaluation of current diagnostic criteria. Obstet Gynecol. Vol. 98, 45-51.

Bergeron, S., Binik, Y. M., Khalifé, S., Pagidas, K., & Glazer, H. I. (2001). Vulvar vestibular syndrome: Rehabilitation of diagnosis and evaluation of current diagnostic criteria. Obstetrics & Gynecology, 98(1), 45-51.

Berghmans, L. C., Hendriks, H. J., Bo, K., Hay-Smith, E. J., de Bie, R. A., & van Waalwijk van Doorn, E. S. (1998). Conservative treatment of stress urinary incontinence in women: A systematic review of randomized clinical trials. British Journal of Urology, 82(2), 181-91.

Berghmans, L., Frederiks, C., de Bie, R., Weil, E., Smeets, L., van Waalwijk van Doorn, E, et al. (1996). Efficacy of biofeedback, when included with pelvic floor muscle exercise treatment, for genuine stress incontinence. Neurology and Urodynamics, 15(1), 37-52.

Block, Jennifer. (2007). Pushed. The Painful Truth About Childbirth and Modern Maternity Care. Cambridge, MA: Da Capo Press.

Butler, D. S. (2004). Mobilisation of the nervous system. Edinborough: Churchill Livingston.

Bo, K., & Sherburn, M. (2005). Evaluation of female pelvic floor muscle function and strength. Physical Therapy, 85(3), 269-282.

Borello-France, D., Zyczynski, H., Downey, P, Rause, C. & Wister, J. (2006). Effect of pelvic-floor muscle exercise position on continence and quality-of-life outcomes in women with stress urinary incontinence. Physical Therapy, 86(7), 974-986.

Bouchez, Colette. (2001). The V Zone: A Woman's Guide to Intimate Health Care. New York, NY: Fireside.

Calais-Germain, Blandine. (2003). The Female Pelvis: Anatomy & Exercises. Seattle, WA: Eastland Press.

Calais-Germain, Blandine. (2005). Anatomy of Breathing. Seattle, WA: Eastland Press.

Calleja-Agius J, Brincat MP. (2009). Urogenital atrophy. Climacteric. Apr 22, pp. 1-7

Carriere, Neate, and Feldt, Cynthia Markel. (2006). The Pelvic Floor. Stuttgart, Germany: Georg Thieme Verlag.

Cauthery, Dr. Philip, Stanway, Dr. Andrew, and Stanway, Dr. Penny. (1983). The Complete Book of Love and Sex. Great Britain: Century Publishing Co. Ltd.

Chu, K. K., Chen, F. P., Chang, S. D., & Soong, Y. K. (1995). Laparoscopic presacral neurectomy in the treatment of dysmenorrhea. Diagnostic and Therapeutic Endoscopy, 1, 223-225.

D'Amborosio, Kerry J, Roth, George B. (1997). Positional Release Therapy, Assessment and Treatment of Musculoskeletal Dysfunction. St. Louis, Missouri: Mosby.

Davies, Clair and Amber Davies. (2004). The Trigger Point Therapy Workbook: Your Self-Treatment Guide for Pain Relief. Oakland, CA: New Harbinger Publications.

Davis, Martha, Ph.D, Robbins-Eshelman, Elizabeth, M.S.W., and McKay, Matthew, Ph.D. (2000). The Relaxation and Stress Reduction Workbook. New York, NY: MJM Books.

Dell, JR, Mokrzycki, ML, Jayne, CJ. (2009). Differentiating interstitial cystitis from similar conditions commonly seen in gynecologic practice. Eur J Obstet Gynecol Reprod Biol. Apr 29.

Dul, Jan and Weerdmeester, Bernard. (2001). Ergonomics for Beginners: A Quick Reference Guide. Second Edition. London: Taylor & Francis.

Dumoulin, C., Lemieux, M., Bourbonnais, D., Gravel, D., Bravo, G. & Morin, M. (2004). Physiotherapy for persistent postnatal stress urinary incontinence: a randomized controlled trial. Obstetrics & Gynecology, 104(3), 504-510.

Dye, J. (2004). Fertility of American Women: June 2004. Current Population Report, December 2005, 1-14.

Ehrstrom S, Kornfeld D, Rylander E, Bohm-Starke N. (2009). Chronic stress in women with localized provoked vulvodynia. J Psychosom Obstet Gynaecol. March Vol. 30(1), pp. 73-9.

Epstein, Abby, and Lake, Ricki. (2009) Your Best Birth. New York, NY: Hachette Book Group.

Fanucci E, Manenti G, Ursone A, Fusco N, Mylonakou I, D'Urso S, Simonetti G. (2009). Role of interventional radiology in pudendal neuralgia: a description of techniques and review of the literature. Radiol Med. Mar 10.

Fisher, K. & Riolo, L. (2004). Evidence in practice. American Physical Therapy Association Inc. Retrieved June 12, 2008 from http://www.thefreelibrary.com/evidence+in+practice-a0120610455.com

FitzGerald, M.P. & Kotarinos, R. (2003). Rehabilitation of the short pelvic floor. I: Background and patient evaluation. International Urogynecological Journal, 14(4), 261-268.

FitzGerald, M.P. & Kotarinos, R. (2003). Rehabilitation of the short pelvic floor. II: Treatment of the patient with the short pelvic floor. International Urogynecological Journal, 14 (4), 269-275.

Franklin, Eric. (2002). Pelvic Power: Mind/Body Exercises for Strength, Flexibility, Posture, and Balance. Hightstown, NJ: Princeton Book Company.

Gerwin, R., Dommerholt, J., & Shah, J. (2004). An explanation of simons' integrated hypothesis of trigger point formation. Current Science Inc., 8, 468-475.

Glazer, H., & MacConkey, D. (1996). Functional rehabilitation of pelvic floor muscles: A challenge to tradition. Urologic Nursing, 16, 68-9. Retrieved May 25, 2008 from http://www.vulvodynia.com/fropfm.htm.

Goldberg, Roger. (2003) Ever Since I Had My Baby: Understanding, Treating, and Preventing the Most Common Physical Aftereffects of Pregnancy and Childbirth. New York: Three Rivers Press.

Goldfinger C, Pukall CF, Gentilcore-Saulnier E, McLean L, Chamberlain S. (2009). A prospective study of pelvic floor physical therapy: Pain and psychosexual outcomes in provoked vestibulodynia. J Sex Med. April 28.

Goldstein, A. (2008). Vulvodynia (CME). J Sex Med. 2008 Jan;5(1):5-15 18173761 Retrieved December 12, 2008, from http://lib.bioinfo.pl/auth:Goldstein,AT.

Goldstein, A. (2007). New diagnosis for vestibular pain and redness: Don't get lumped in a general category again! OurGyn. Retrieved February 12, 2009, from http://www.ourgyn.com.

Goldstein, A. (2007). Vaginal pain and itching with no known cause? OurGyn. Retrieved February 21, 2009, from http://www.ourgyn.com.

Goldstein, A. (2007). 14 different treatments for vulvar vestibulitis syndrome. OurGyn. Retrieved May 23, 2008 from http://www.ourgyn.com/content/index.php?option=com_content&task=view&id=18&Itemid=66.

Goldfinger, S. (2007). Gas and bloating. UpToDate. Retrieved July 11, 2008, from http://www.uptodate.com/patients/content/topic.do?topicKey=~ S6QjVerp-W9eT4.

Haefner, H., Collins, M., Davis, G., Edwards, L., Foster, D., Hartmann, E., et al (2005). The Vulvodynia Guideline. Journal of Lower Genital Tract Disease, 9(1), 40-51.

Harlow, B., & Stewart, E. (2003). A population-based assessment of chronic unexplained vulvar pain: Have we underestimated the prevalence of vulvodynia? Journal of the American Medical Women's Association, 58(2), 82-87.

Haslam, Jeanette, and Laycock, Jo. (2002). Therapeutic Management of Incontinence and Pelvic Pain. Second Edition. London, England: Springer-Verlag.

Hay, Louise L. (1999). You Can Heal Your Life. Carlsbad, CA: Hay House Inc.

Hopwood, Val, and Lovesey, Maureen, and Mokone, Sara. (1997). Acupuncture & Related Techniques in Physical Therapy. Edinburgh, England: Churchill Livingstone.

Hulme, Janet A. (1997) Beyond Kegels. Second Edition. Missoula, MT: Phoenix Publishing Co.

Hutcherson, Hilda. (2002). What Your Mother Never Told You About S-e-x. New York, NY: Berkley Publishing Group.

Jones, L. H., Kusunose, R. H. & Goering, E. K. (1995). Jones Strain-Counterstrain. Boise, ID: Jones Strain-Counterstrain Inc.

Kabatt-Zin, Jon. (2005). Coming to Our Senses. New York, New York: Hyperion.

Katz, Ditza and Ross Lynn Tabisel. (2005). Private Pain: Understanding Vaginismus & Dyspareunia. Second Edition. Canada: Katz-Tabi Publications.

Kavaler, Elizabeth. (2006). A Seat on the Aisle, Please: The Essential Guide To Urinary Tract Problems in Women. New York, NY: Copernicus Books.

Kellogg-Spadt, S., & Albaugh, J. (2002). Intimacy and bladder pain: helping women reclaim sexuality. Urologic Nursing, 22(5), 355-56.

Kellogg-Spadt, S., & Giordano, J. (2002). Vulvar Vestibulitis and Sexual Pain. The Female Patient, 27, 51-53.

Klein, M., & Robbins, R. (1998). Let me count the ways (Discovering great sex without intercourse). New York, NY: Penguin Putnam Inc.

KMom (2003). Pelvic pain (Symphysis publis dysfunction). Retrieved August 14, 2008, from http://www.plus-size-pregnancy.org/pubicpain.htm.

Lachowsky M, Nappi R. (2009). The effects of estrogen on urogenital health. Maturitas. April 30.

Lee, R. B., Stone, K., Magelssen, D., Belts, R. P., & Benson, W. L. (1986). Presacral neurectomy for chronic pelvic pain. Obstetrics & Gynecology, 68, 517-521. Retrieved April 17, 2008, from http://www.greenjournal.org/cgi/content/abstract/68/4/517.

Levin-Gervasi, Stephanie. (1995). The Back Pain Sourcebook. Los Angeles, CA: Lowell House.

Magee, David J. (2002). Orthopedic Physical Assessment. Philadelphia, PA: Saunders Publications.

Makichen, Walter. (2005). Spirit Babies. How to Communicate with the Child

You're Meant to Have. New York, NY Bantam Dell.

Manheim, Carol. (2001). The Myofascial Release Manual. Third Edition. Thorofare, NJ: Slack Inc.

Mercier, Patricia. (2007). The Chakra Bible. New York, NY: Sterling Publishing.

Miller, P., Forstein, D. & Styles, S. (2008). Effect of short-term diet and exercise on hormone levels and menses in obese, infertile women. Journal of Reproductive Medicine, 53(5), 315-319.

Mojay, Gabriel. (1997). Aromatherapy for Healing the Spirit: Restoring Emotional and Mental Balance with Essential Oils. Rochester, Vermont: Healing Arts Press.

Moldwin, R. (2000). The interstitial cystitis survival guide: Your guide to the latest treatment options and coping strategies. Oakland, CA: New Harbinger Publications.

Morkved, S., Bo, K. & Fjortoft, T. (2002). Effect of adding biofeedback to pelvic floor muscle training to treat urodynamic stress incontinence. Obstetrics & Gynecology, 100(4), 730-739.

Myers, Thomas W. (2001). Anatomy Trains. Myofascial Meridians and Movement Therapists. Edinburgh, England: Churchill Livingstone.

Netter, Frank H. (1989). Atlas of Human Anatomy. Teterboro, New Jersey. Icon Learning Systems.

Neumann, Donald A. (2002). Kinesiology of the Musculoskeletal System: Foundations or Physical Rehabilitation. St. Louis: Mosby Inc.

Newman, D. (2008). Understanding electrical stimulation as a treatment for incontinence. Seekwellness. Retrieved January 14, 2009, from http://www.seekwellness.com/incontinence/electric_stim.htm.

Noble, Elizabeth. (1995). Essential Exercises for the Childbearing Year. Harwich, MA: New Life Images.

Prendergast, S., & Weiss, J. (2003). Screening for musculoskeletal causes of pelvic pain. Clinical Obstetrics & Gynecology, 46(4), 1-10.

Rao, S. (2004). Diagnosis and management of fecal incontinence. The American Journal of Gastroenterology, 99(8), 1585-1604.

Rogers, Rebecca G, Janet Yagoda Shagam and Shelley Kleinschmidt. (2006). Regaining Bladder Control: What Every Woman Needs to Know. New York, NY: Prometheus Books.

Sapsford, R., & Hodges, P. (2001). Contraction of the pelvic floor muscles during abdominal maneuvers. Archives of Physical Medicine and Rehabilitation, 82(8), 1081-8.

Sapsford Aua, Ruth et al. (1998) Women's Health: A Textbook for Physiotherapist. New York: WB Saunders Company Ltd.

Sapsford, R. (2001). "Contraction of the pelvic floor muscles during abdominal maneuvers." Abstract: Arch Phys Med Rehabil. Vol. 81, 1081-8.

Schnaubet, Kurt. (1999). Medical Aromatherapy. Healing with Essential Oils. Berkely, CA: Frog, Ltd.

Shamliyan, T., Kane, R., Wyman, J. & Wilt, T. (2008). Systematic review: randomized, controlled trials of nonsurgical treatments for urinary incontinence in women. Annals of Internal Medicine, 148(6), 459-473.

Spadt-Kellogg, S.,et al. (2002). Vulvar Vestibulitis and sexual pain: New insights. The Female Patient. Vol. 27, 51-53.

Spadt-Kellogg, Susan, et al. (2002). Intimacy and bladder pain: Helping women reclaim sexuality. Urologic Nursing Vol. 22:5, 355-56.

Spatafora, Denise. (2009). Better Birth. Hoboken, New Jersey: Wiley and Sons, Inc.

Steege JF, Zolnoun DA. (2009). Evaluation and treatment of dyspareunia. Obstet Gynecol. May 113(5), pp. 1124-36.

Steward, Elizabeth G. and Paula Spencer. (2002). The V Book: A Doctor's Guide to Complete Vulvovaginal Health. New York, NY: Bantam Books.

Sutton KS, Pukall CF, Chamberlain S. (2009). Pain ratings, sensory thresholds, and psychosocial functioning in women with provoked vestibulodynia. J Sex Marital Ther. Vol. 35(4), pp. 262-81.

Tjaden, B., Schlaff, W. D., Kimball, A., & Rock, J. A. (1990). The efficacy of presacral neurectomy for the relief of midline dysmenorrhea. Obstetrics & Gynecology, 76, 89-91. Retrieved February 13, 2008, from http://www.greenjournal.org/cgi/content/abstract/76/1/89.

Tolle, Eckhart. (1999). The Power of Now. Vancouver, Canada: Namaste Publishing.

Wallace, Kathe and Holly Herman. (2006). Female Pelvic Floor: Function, Dysfunction and Treatment. Level 2B. The Prometheus Group: Secaucus, NJ, Nov 3-5 2006.

Wallace, Kathe and Holly Herman. (2007). Female Pelvic Floor: Function, Dysfunction and Treatment. Level 3. The Prometheus Group: New York, NY, May 4-6 2007.

Wallace, Kathe and Holly Herman. (2008). Female Pelvic Floor: Function, Dysfunction and Treatment. Level 1. The Prometheus Group: Hunter College, March 7-9 2008.

Weiss, J. (2000). Chronic pelvic pain and myofascial trigger points. The Pain Clinic, 13(6), 13-18.

Weiss, J. (2001). Pelvic floor myofascial trigger point: Manual therapy for interstitial cystitis and the urgency-frequency syndrome. The Journal of Urology, 166(6), 2226-2231.

Weiss, J. (2003). Pudendal nerve entrapment. Presented at the International Pelvic Pain Society 10th Scientific Meeting of Chronic Pelvic Pain in Alberta, Canada August 2003, 1-25.

Wetzler, Gail, PT. (2009). Gynecologic Visceral Manipulation. Alexandria, VA: American Physical Therapy Association.

Wise, D. & Anderson, R. (2003). A headache in the pelvis: A new understanding and treatment for chronic pelvic pain syndromes. Occidental, CA: National Center for Pelvic Pain.

Worwood, Valerie Ann. (1996). The Fragrant Mind. Aromatherapy for Personality, Mind, and Emotion. Novato, CA: New World Library.

Index

11198417R0